P9-EDW-149

Health Promotion
Ideas That **Work**

POINT LOMA NAZARENE UNIVERSITY
RYAN LIBRARY
3900 LOMALAND DRIVE
SAN DIEGO, CALIFORNIA 92106-2899

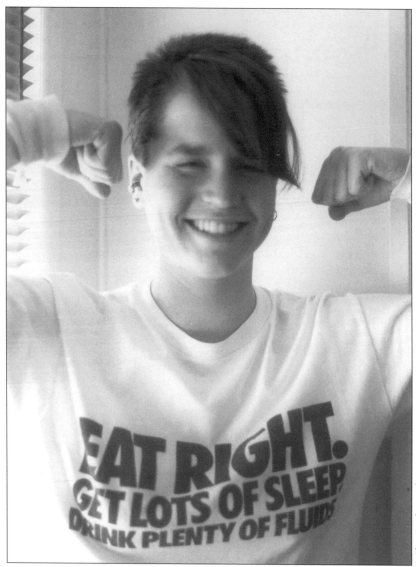

© Cleo Freelance Photo

613
G547h
6/02

Health Promotion Ideas That **Work**

Timothy E. Glaros, MA

Creative Business Consulting
Grey Eagle, MN

POINT LOMA NAZARENE UNIVERSITY
WITHDRAWN
RYAN LIBRARY

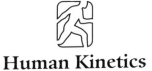

Human Kinetics

Library of Congress Cataloging-in-Publication Data

Glaros, Timothy E., 1945-
   Health promotion ideas that work / Timothy E. Glaros.
     p. cm.
   ISBN 0-87322-888-X
   1. Health promotion.   I. Title.
RA427.8.G53 1997
613--dc21

97-9584
CIP

ISBN: 0-87322-888-X

Copyright © 1997 by Timothy E. Glaros

All rights reserved. Except for use in a review, the reproduction or utilization of this work in any form or by any electronic, mechanical, or other means, now known or hereafter invented, including xerography, photocopying, and recording, and in any information storage and retrieval system, is forbidden without the written permission of the publisher.

Acquisitions Editors: Rick Frey and Scott Wikgren; **Developmental Editor:** Kristine Enderle; **Assistant Editors:** Coree Schutter and Tony Callihan; **Editorial Assistant:** Laura Ward Majersky; **Copyeditor:** Jacqueline Eaton Blakley; **Proofreader:** Erin Cler; **Graphic Designer:** Keith Blomberg; **Graphic Artist:** Kim McFarland; **Photo Editor:** Boyd LaFoon; **Cover Designer:** Jack Davis; **Printer:** Versa Press

Printed in the United States of America   10 9 8 7 6 5 4 3

Human Kinetics
Web site: www.humankinetics.com

United States: Human Kinetics, P.O. Box 5076, Champaign, IL 61825-5076
1-800-747-4457
e-mail: humank@hkusa.com

Canada: Human Kinetics, 475 Devonshire Road, Unit 100, Windsor, ON N8Y 2L5
1-800-465-7301 (in Canada only)
e-mail: humank@hkcanada.com

Europe: Human Kinetics, P.O. Box IW14, Leeds LS16 6TR, United Kingdom
+44 (0)113-278 1708
e-mail: humank@hkeurope.com

Australia: Human Kinetics, 57A Price Avenue, Lower Mitcham, South Australia 5062
(08) 82771555
e-mail: liahka@senet.com.au

New Zealand: Human Kinetics, P.O. Box 105-231, Auckland Central
09-309-1890
e-mail: humank@hknewz.com

DEDICATION

This book is dedicated to the memory of my brother Ted Glaros, who was my coach, mentor, and friend.

And to the healthy futures of Stephanie, Sunni, and Ben.

CONTENTS

PREFACE

Health Promotion Ideas That Work is based on the popular presentations I have delivered across the country to health promotion organizations such as the Association for Worksite Health Promotion (AWHP) and the Wellness Councils of America (WELCOA). My presentations offer program themes and concepts that can be applied in most health promotion settings with a few modifications. The presentations cover the full range of interest areas and core program activities, and incorporate audience input to modify and improve those ideas as well as to create and share additional ideas.

In this book, I have organized these activity ideas by health topics. This organization allows you to quickly and easily find activities that support your program goals. You can then concentrate on implementation and meeting the needs of your population rather than getting bogged down in the often difficult process of devising program concepts. *Health Promotion Ideas That Work* is sure to become one of your most used resources.

Health promotion programs across the country are being conducted by several different types of professionals with two common characteristics—they have limited resources and they have a passion for their assignments. One group includes those whose primary responsibility is something other than health promotion, such as human resources or occupational health. These individuals are faced with the challenge of planning and implementing an important program for their organization with minimal formal training and a limited network within the health promotion field. A second group is comprised of people who are trained in the field but are greatly overextended and without a continuous supply of creative stimulation because they work alone. A third group contains those with a high level of technical training in a health-related field but limited talent in promotion. A fourth group includes college students preparing for a career in health promotion. If you fall into one of these groups and are in search of easy-to-administer, inexpensive program ideas, this book is designed for you. The purpose of this book is to assist you by providing a wealth of health promotion program ideas that are creative and easy to implement. These ideas will enhance any program and simplify the planning process while significantly improving participation.

In order to make your job easier, I have tried to make this book as user-friendly as possible. Some ideas have been included without extensive detail when it seemed clear that they would need to be modified from their original format due to their local specificity. Others are so generic that they can be used with little or no modification. In many cases, the idea I present will stimulate your own creativity and send you in a totally new direction.

Many of the ideas will be easier to implement if you obtain materials from one or more appropriate resources. In some cases you will find it essential because the idea is built on a specific product or service. To this end, I have included a list of some useful resources in an appendix at the end of the book. I have listed mailing addresses, phone and fax numbers, e-mail addresses, and web addresses whenever possible. I encourage you to develop an extensive database and hard-copy file system of the materials from these and other resources that you encounter. Many of these resources will become additional sources of new ideas since that may be part of their mission. Take advantage of the free catalogs and sample materials that many of them offer. Stay on their mailing lists so you will be informed as new programs and ideas are developed.

So take out your plan for the coming 12 months and start browsing the text. Look for major activities that will need special promotional efforts to achieve your participation goals. Look at any idea that is even remotely associated with your activity and use it as a jumping off point. Use the techniques described in chapter 1 and you will be well on the way to a more successful health promotion program.

ACKNOWLEDGMENT

The author wishes to thank Vivian Neiger for helping him get unstuck whenever he needed it.

Health Promotion Ideas

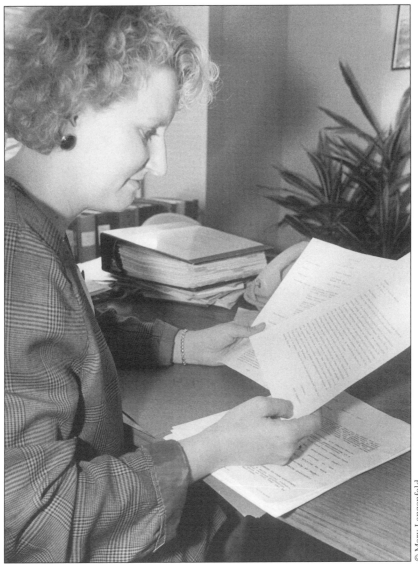

© Mary Langenfeld

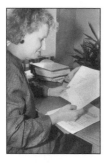

Producing creative ideas is one of the most rewarding and challenging tasks of a health promotion professional. The process is easiest for those of us who have the luxury of working in large organizations with many colleagues, as brainstorming is generally more efficient and productive in a group setting. However, most of us find ourselves working alone on these projects, relying on our own ingenuity to fuel the creative process. Therefore, the purpose of this text is to share ideas that have been created by others. Many of them can be used as presented, while others may be modified or may serve as catalysts for your own program ideas.

This chapter outlines a system that will help you develop your own ideas, particularly when you don't have anyone to help stimulate the creative process. This system consists of several distinct steps:

- Find your starting point
- Plant the seeds of your idea
- Research your idea
- Develop your program

Several strategies can be applied within this system to enhance the creative process.

Find Your Starting Point

The first step in creating a health promotion idea that works is to determine a starting point. The starting point will give you a framework for the subsequent steps. The three most common starting points are the topic, the timing, and the target population. These three starting points will often interact with each other as the idea develops.

Topic

Topic refers to the subject area addressed by the program. Topics come in all shapes and sizes. Common ones include nutrition, walking, and self-care. These starting points can fuel development of your ideas and serve as a catalyst for determining other concepts like the promotional activity, theme, title, and graphics. For example, titles such as *Walktoberfest* or a theme such as *Walk a Mall in Your Shoes* built upon the starting point topic of walking. Thoroughly examine all aspects of the topic when searching for a starting point so that you don't overlook better possibilities.

Timing

The second starting point is the timing of the event—that is, the time of year, season, month, or special day when the event is scheduled. Timing influences the direction of your idea. For example, you would *Swing Into Summer* during the spring or early summer months of May and June, or *Declare Your Independence From Smoking* on July 4th as the country celebrates Independence Day.

Virtually any day of the year contains possibilities for creative promotions. Carefully consider the day, month, season, and all the concepts associated with each of these as you determine the starting point.

Target Population

Determining specific characteristics of your target population is an excellent starting point. This usually increases the appeal of your activity, and therefore the odds of your target group attending. Characteristics that you should consider include age, sex, job type, educational level, income level, and marital status.

Any of these characteristics can, either alone or in combination, help you determine your target population's special interests, learning styles, preferences, or other factors that will influence your program. Using these differences allows you to divide your total eligible population into "market segments." Market segments are subsets of the larger group that share common characteristics. When you are designing a promotion you can then take the common characteristics into consideration. This will increase the likelihood that you will reach the participants you are targeting.

For example, imagine that your target population includes a large segment of middle-aged employees. Knowing that this age group is considered the "sandwich generation," you could design special programming to address issues of concern to them such as elder care and adult children living at home. And your awareness of the concerns of most in this age group regarding financial retirement planning could lead you to offer training programs on this subject. As you plan fitness classes, you could choose to offer a class to address the specific fitness needs of middle-aged employees. If you determine that many of these middle-aged employees are women, a seminar on menopause is likely to be a popular and helpful offering.

When designing separate programs for men and women, you could consider what appeals to a specific sex in aerobics classes and differing goals in weight training. Or design activities that address gender-based health concerns, such as seminars that address prostate cancer or breast cancer.

Your long-range planning may have revealed differences in perceived stress among people with different job types. You may have noticed that a specific group has a legitimate excuse for not participating in your programs due to their work schedule. Or you may have had requests for travel stress programs for those employees who travel extensively.

Having a starting point and knowing the details of your target population is the foundation for your health promotion idea. You are now ready to develop the idea further.

Plant the Seeds of Your Idea

Once you have determined a starting point for an idea, you need to begin to give it some focus. At this point, the activity may or may not have developed in your mind. In either case, you can take the creative process to the next stage by developing a central theme or concept that captures the essence of your intention. Often the concept or theme will jump right out at you. If it does not, you can use your wellness committee or the employee population at large to assist you in the process.

Determining a Theme or Concept

When developing a theme, expand on the starting point by using many of the resources at your disposal—like your thoughts, your wellness committee, or your would-be participants.

Using Your Thoughts for Ideas.   Toss around the program idea in your head awhile. Start developing the title by using alliteration, acronyms, or maybe even a play on words.

An alliteration is a phrase with the same letter, word, or sound repeated in all the key words. For example, some catchy titles might be:

- *Fitness at Fifty* (modified fitness course)
- *Menopause Myths* (seminar)
- *Care for the Caregivers* (elder care series)
- *Secretarial Stress* (brown-bag luncheon)
- *Vital Vitamins* (nutrition-related newsletter article)

Another good trick is to use an acronym, a single word whose letters are comprised of the first letters of the words of a clever phrase. For example:

- *Put G.A.S. on the Fire* (Great American Smokeout)
- *Join the F.A.T. Exercise Program* (Fit and Trim)

- *S.O.S. Information Series* (Stamp Out Stress)

You can also use a play on words by twisting or stretching the meaning of a word in an unusual or clever way. For example:

- *Bone Up on Osteoporosis* (seminar series about risk factors for osteoporosis)
- *Muscle Your Way Into Fitness* (exercise program that focuses on strength training)
- *People Kneading People* (seminar for upper-body partner massage)

Frequently you will not be able to devise a clever theme or concept. You may have to settle for a very succinct description of the activity such as *Long-Range Retirement Planning* or *Last-Minute Retirement Planning* for retirement planning seminars, or *Dance Aerobics* and *Sport Aerobics* as descriptors for classes designed to attract women or men.

Plain, clear descriptions for health promotion activities are not necessarily bad or ineffective, they are just not as much fun. However, on some occasions a fun title is not appropriate—for example, programs dealing with AIDS education or coping with grief.

Using Your Wellness Committee for Ideas.   One difficulty you face if you work alone is that of generating or maintaining creative energy. Creative energy seems to be maximized by group interaction. If you find yourself in this position and feel "blocked" on idea formation and development, include your wellness committee in the creative process.

Make one of the agenda items for a given meeting the formation or development of a promotion idea. You could include a brainstorming session as part of your meeting agenda on a regular basis. Sometimes you might need to use regular sessions for broader, less focused planning.

It might help to conduct a training session on the creative process to introduce the group to creative techniques or identify members of the committee who have a particular knack for creativity.

Be sure to reward your committee appropriately and give them credit for their contributions. Their participation will enhance your efforts and provide additional employee ownership for the program.

Using Participants for Ideas.   A second source of group energy is the general employee population. Every workplace is bound to have creative individuals with a flair for the unusual. Many of them will not necessarily be part of your wellness committee. Others will have a strong desire to contribute but will not have the time to commit to a formal committee assignment.

However, you can recruit creative employees with many methods. For instance, hold a competition for new ideas. The most obvious example is the typical "name the program" contest used when new programs are being started.

Another way to get assistance in the idea development process is to set up a short-term committee or task force. First, put out a company-wide call for volunteers for a particular program. If the response is insufficient, scan your participant lists from previous classes, clubs, and other activities for individuals who appear to have a special interest in the topic you are trying to develop. Approach them individually with a request for assistance.

If you don't want to create a formal committee, recruit one or two individuals. Look for people who are known for a good sense of humor or creativity. This may even be their point of entry into participation in the program.

Be sure that all of your requests make it clear that the assignment is short-term in nature. Remember that commitment may be what has kept many of these employees from offering their assistance thus far.

Using Your Megalist for Ideas.   Often the most creative ideas come to us at times when we have no use for them. However, something inside tells us that the idea has merit—not now, but at some time in the future. Many of these ideas may not ever become programs, but will serve as a starting point or stimulant for other program ideas. Begin creating a *megalist* by recording enough information about some of your successful ideas to allow you to recycle them in the future. Then add ideas you feel have merit but you don't have an opportunity to use in the near future. Add seeds of ideas such as a clever theme or simple concept. Capture these thoughts so they don't slip away, and develop them later. Build on this list over time and do some simple classification to allow easy retrieval. If you begin thinking of yourself as a creative idea person, you will be surprised at how many ideas come to you from a large variety of sources.

Research Your Idea

Once you have a central theme or concept in place, you can move to the next step—researching the idea. Don't be surprised, however, if you have inadvertently stumbled across many pieces of information at this point. You may even have a very solid notion of the entire promotional plan by this time. However, if you have the time, it is worthwhile to do some research. Your goal is to gather, in no particular order, as many thoughts, connections, facts, and other information as can be incorporated into the program. Some good sources of information include:

- Calendars
- Other programs
- Your old ideas
- Media events
- Networking

Calendars

The calendar can be a source of information that is useful to the development of an idea. If you have determined in advance that the event should occur on a specific day or during a specific week, you should examine the calendar for that period of time to see if any historical information pertains to your event. In particular, look for anniversaries that occur on the dates in question. Also consult *Chase's Calendar of Events* for data (see the appendix, page 130). Every day of the year has some special designation bestowed by some government body or special-interest group. Alternatively, you might find an appropriate day in the calendar that will then drive the timing of the event. For example, in the process of planning a swimming exercise journey across the English Channel, examining the calendar will reveal several anniversaries of crossings by swimmers. (This event does not entail physically swimming the English Channel—you'll read more about exercise journeys in chapter 2.) You will also find the dates of the Normandy invasion and the completion of the tunnel between England and France. This data gives you several choices for timing the event. Depending on the choice you make, you can then research details about the event associated with the date you chose and incorporate that information into the planning.

Other Programs

Additional information useful in fully developing an idea can be found in other health promotion programs. You may have encountered an idea implemented by another program in another part of the country, perhaps part of a poster presentation or luncheon conversation at a conference or other professional meeting. The idea as implemented by the other program may have been the conscious or unconscious source of your idea. In many cases, the basic structure of the idea may contain the majority of the information you need, but would not work in your region. For example, the *Hollywood Stars* weight-control activity described in chapter 6 (Promotion #37) may have originated in Southern California, but using the names of professional sports personalities may be more effective if you are in a major professional sports city. Or winter themes may need to be modified if they were implemented in the North but you are in the South. In any case, if the idea has characteristics similar to yours, researching the other program may provide a wealth of information useful to your project.

Your Old Ideas

Another source of valuable information is your files of old ideas that you may have implemented in the past. An idea may have fizzled the first time around yet has components that still have merit, such as graphics or incentive strategies. An example of using previously implemented ideas is the *Conquering Mount Everest and Other Lofty Pursuits* stairclimbing event (Promotion #12, chapter 4). The first time through you may have done everything but use climbing teams. If you kept notes as part of your evaluation, you would have the information recommending the use of teams. Knowing this, your next mountain climb could use all of the same steps but add the use of teams. You may, however, choose a different date to coincide with another mountain's ascension anniversary, especially if you live in a mountainous area and can choose a local peak. Researching your old program notes will give you plenty of data to help you plan your current event.

Media Events

Anticipating the probable events promoted by various media can be another source of information for planning. This is particularly true when your event is built around a nationally recognized day, week, or month. For example, if you are putting together activities for National Heart Month, you can obtain information from the American Heart Association about local media coverage. They may also be able to share information about national coverage. Calls to your local television stations, radio stations, and newspapers may also give you ideas. If you are particularly persuasive and have a program with human interest, you may even be able to get some local coverage of your event. This level of visibility will give a very positive boost to your program and event. It can give the program increased credibility with nonparticipants, management, and the community at large.

You can also use the media as a rich source of ideas by becoming a student of advertising. Advertising agencies are paid millions of dollars to create ad campaigns that promote use of their client company's products or services. This is no different than what you are trying to accomplish, except that you don't have the resources they do. Scan ads in popular magazines, observe television ads, see what catches your eye on billboards. Try to determine what it is that makes an advertising campaign effective. Borrow techniques as well as the core ideas themselves. Be aware of potential copyright infringement possibilities that would put you and your company at risk before you go too far with an existing idea.

Networking

The final area to be discussed as a source of planning information is that of proactive networking within the health promotion community. If you are in need of new thoughts and perspectives, or are looking for information from other programs, try networking. Get out your professional directory and stack of business cards and begin calling your colleagues. Before making the first call, however, have a specific set of questions ready so you will not forget any important questions and will be respectful of your colleagues' time. Some questions you might consider include:

- Have you ever offered an event similar to this one? (Describe it in general or specific terms.)
- How did you evaluate it? Was it a success?
- What would you do again? Not do again?
- What would you change?
- Do you have any sample materials (flyers, graphics, outlines, handouts, and so forth) you would be willing to share?
- Do you know of any other health promotion professionals who have tried something similar to this?
- Do you have any related ideas that may prove useful?

You will find most professionals very willing to share their ideas, and they will be flattered by your use of their ideas. Be sure to give them credit for their contributions when the opportunity presents itself and be willing to share your programs in return.

Develop Your Program

Now that you have a starting point, a central theme or framework, and sufficient data for your idea, you are ready to complete the idea development process. The next steps are combining the elements and creating an appropriate sequence.

Combining the Elements

The elements of your new idea will consist of all facts, dates, catch phrases, incentives, methods of tracking, graphics ideas, and so on that you have either created or discovered through your research.

You might have enough information to require a system of organization to help you process it. Depending on the complexity and quantity of the elements, begin by organizing them into categories. This may be done with lists on paper or with index cards. The categories will vary with the specific idea, but using weight control as an example, some possibilities include:

- A list of themes such as *Weight a Minute, Weigh to Go,* and *Weight a While*
- A list of dates or holidays that may have significance—for example, Fat Tuesday, Thanksgiving, the anniversary of the invention of the bathroom scale, or New Year's Day
- A list of incentives, such as chances in a drawing for a digital scale or coupons for low-calorie grocery items
- A list of names of people associated either with weight control, overweight, or fitness—for example, King Henry VIII, Jane Fonda, or Oprah Winfrey
- Specific activities such as body composition measurement, logging fat intake, weekly weigh-ins, and partner check-ins
- Anything else that is even a remote possibility for use in the activity

The next step is to evaluate the elements and select those that fit together and best support the idea. You may have chosen a theme of *Weight a Minute,* and combined it with a one-minute weigh-in at lunchtime, a short-term goal built around New Year's resolutions, and salad bar coupons as incentive items. Once you have selected all of the elements, you are ready to assemble them into an appropriate sequence.

Creating an Appropriate Sequence

This is often the final planning step, with one exception. At any time during the creative process, you might have a flash of genius that introduces a new element or moves the idea in a slightly different direction. By all means, pay attention to your instincts in these cases and give serious consideration to incorporating the new idea. On the other hand, when assembling the elements and coordinating them into a logical sequence, you may have a nagging feeling that the plan is somehow imperfect. You may then have to give the idea additional incubation time or a jump start with some specific creative processes to create some new elements.

Arranging the elements will often be very simple with clear logical progressions. Some of the logical points in the sequence include obtaining approval for the overall event plan, and finalizing details that need approval such as the promotion of the event or activity, the registration system, and the core activities of the event.

Obtaining Approval for the Plan.   In our zeal to create the perfect health promotion program, we often get very creative and cross the line between good and bad taste. In most settings, health promotion activities will have to be approved before implementation. The classic example is "potty postings," posters with motivational messages that are posted on the inside doors of lavatory stalls. While these can be extremely effective, in some more formal business settings they may not be considered appropriate. If you are not required to get approval for all activities, run the idea by a sample of your population, management, or the wellness committee before moving ahead. You may also have to obtain approval for certain logistical details such as room reservations or audiovisual equipment.

Promoting the Activity.   All activities need some level of promotion in order to succeed. Even the promotion itself may need its own promotion. For example, if a body composition test is used as a brown-bag luncheon to promote a larger weight-control activity, you must promote the luncheon to get as many people to attend as possible because those are the people likely to attend the larger activity. You will need to consider all the basic concepts of communications and analyze the most effective methods used at your workplace in deciding how to promote the event. Be sure to have some contingency plans for repromotion if initial registration is low. Canceling activities for lack of participation can be very detrimental to a health promotion program. Promotional activities include flyers, bulletin boards, e-mail, newsletter articles, banners, and other communication vehicles.

Throughout the process of developing your idea, you should be on the lookout for appropriate graphics for use with flyers, bulletin boards, incentives, and any other visible component of the activity. Catchy graphics can make a difference in participation, especially with fence-sitters. Purchasing appropriate clip art catalogs either in hard copy or on disk is usually a good investment.

Registration Systems.   Not all activities will need preregistration. However, as part of even the most basic evaluation systems, participation must be tracked. Creating interest lists is an important part of programming that is very useful for follow-up activities as well as evaluation. Preregistration strategies should be built into all promotion that precedes the event. Timing is important if you will be purchasing materials or scheduling instructors based on the response. You must have enough lead time to allow for cancellations, scheduling overflow sessions, or creating and communicating a waiting list response. Attempt to make preregistration as simple as possible in order to eliminate it as a barrier to participation.

If preregistration is not required, then some method of obtaining participants' names and other information should be employed. The simplest method is the traditional "sign up for a free drawing" method used at trade shows, state fairs, and similar events. Create a simple drawing slip requesting the basic information you need and instruct participants to fill it out for a chance in the drawing. Following the weight-control example above, weekly weigh-ins can be submitted on drawing slips each week. This will provide you with an accurate participation list and also encourage compliance with the weigh-in schedule.

The Core Activities.   The next element in the sequence is usually the activity itself. This may consist of several activities in a logical sequence. Using the weight-control example, the first activity could be a brown-bag luncheon pinch test or infrared body composition measurement. The second event could be a one-hour seminar on body composition where in-depth information on the topic is shared. The third event could be a six-week body composition enhancement class where participants employ nutrition, weight-control, and fitness skills to attempt to reduce their percent body fat.

You're Ready!

You are now ready to create program ideas that work in any setting. With the program ideas to come in chapters 3 through 10, you have an extensive list of ideas that have been used by other professionals as well as a process for developing more of your own. Remember that none of the ideas presented in this book should be considered perfect or complete when applied to your unique situation. Use the creative processes described in this chapter to modify the ideas found in the remaining chapters of the book. Be sure to keep notes and files on your ideas and share them with others in the field. Take advantage of the many sources of information and assistance available from the resources listed in the appendix. Build your own database of additional resources as you discover them.

Since creativity is not only an essential element of a successful health promotion program but also is one of the most satisfying elements to incorporate into your job, it seems appropriate that you as a health promotion professional continue to improve your creative skills. By doing so, you will continually improve your programs and your job satisfaction. Plus, these skills will become useful in other aspects of your life and will become a part of your job skills just as computer skills or public speaking may have. Apply your creativity and the techniques described in this chapter to enhance your planning process. This will give you some immediate and direct practice with the skills, as well as moving the program ideas to a higher level. Put your creative energy to work and enjoy helping others to make the lifestyle changes that will make their lives more enjoyable, productive, and healthy.

CHAPTER 2

Useful Program Concepts

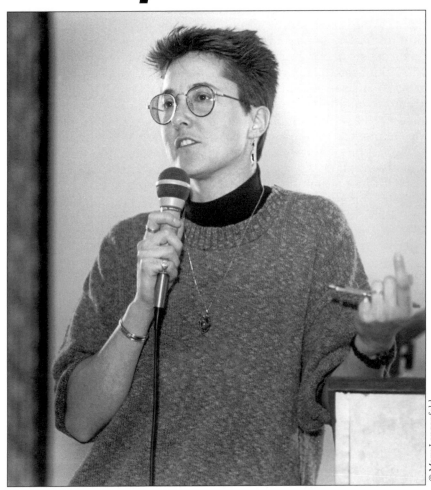

© Mary Langenfeld

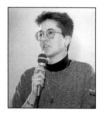

Health promotion programs and activities are comprised of two distinct components—the health component and the promotion component. Most of us are well-versed in the health component, having college degrees ranging from general health education or health promotion to highly specialized technical expertise such as nutrition or exercise physiology. Most of us, however, are not as well-versed in the promotional component, which is more akin to marketing and advertising than education. It is the promotional aspect of our programs that provides the gateway to the health education, health interventions, and lifestyle changes we hope to bring to our participants. Our ability to attract participants through promotional efforts is therefore a major determinant of our overall success in health promotion. The activities described in the following chapters are offered with the hope that they will supplement the technical knowledge we bring to the profession and increase our effectiveness.

Health promotion ideas in this book will be categorized according to their promotion type. For the sake of clarity in the following chapters, a few definitions of terms used in the text will be useful. The four program promotion concepts include:

 Monthly Minutes

 Exercise Journeys

 Seminar Series

 Theme Events

Monthly Minutes

Monthly Minutes are brief promotional events that have four general characteristics. First, they should take very little time—in most cases, literally a minute. Second, they should have an educational or informational component, if only a few facts. Third, they should have a promotional component; that is, they are not events in themselves, but rather promote a higher level of health promotion activity such as a more lengthy promotion or an extensive health education class. Fourth, they should include a written handout for participants to take away. The handout could include information, recipes, or self-tests, and often will have some form of activity registration.

Monthly Minutes are particularly well-suited for use in cafeteria and health fair settings. They are also generally very low-cost and often can be administered by volunteers from the employee population or public agencies. The brief meetings offer a unique opportunity for informal and fun face-to-face interaction with your participants, helping to personalize your programs. You will find that Monthly Minutes offer a low-risk, low-commitment point of entry for many employees who are reluctant to begin affiliating with the program at higher levels.

Exercise Journeys

Exercise journeys is a term that categorizes the myriad of activities that involve walking, running, or swimming to a predetermined destination. That is, participants track the amount of time or miles they spend in a physical activity, and that time or distance is applied to an imaginary journey. They include walks across America, mountain climbing on stairs, stationary bike tours, and similar events. Beyond the basic definition, a couple of examples will be described in more detail for those professionals who may not be familiar with the design of these programs.

The basis of designing an exercise journey is to first select either a "trip" that has historical significance (such as the anniversary of the conquest of Mount Everest), a destination of general interest (such as going to New Orleans in time for Mardi Gras), or a destination of local significance (such as a tour of your company's major customers' locations or your own satellite offices). You will need to gather some basic information about this destination or goal, like the distance from your location to the destination, height of the mountain, or exact date of the anniversary.

You will then need to make some estimates of the amount and type of physical activity needed to accomplish the goal. For example, if you were going to walk to a destination that is 300 miles away, and your average fitness walker covered 2 miles per day and walked 5 days per week, you can estimate that it would take one participant 30 weeks to complete the journey. In order to maintain interest on an exercise journey, a time span of six to eight weeks is recommended to complete the event. This then means that organizing the event into "exercise buddies" consisting of two participants per team would take 15 weeks if you combine their mileage, 10 weeks if you organized groups of three, or 6 weeks for groups of five walkers.

Other ways of adjusting the mileage include using aerobic conversions based on minutes of exercise; for example, an hour of swimming could certainly be given distance credit equivalent to an hour of walking or running. The important aspect of the conversion is to allow all exercisers to participate and have reasonably equitable conversions so that all can complete the activity within your time constraints. Using highly visible graphics on an easel or bulletin board makes these activities more fun for participants, especially if they can see their names in print. Use maps or diagrams to graphically chart progress on these journeys.

Seminar Series

A *seminar series* is exactly what it sounds like—a series of single-session educational presentations. All seminars in the series should be related to each other but should also be able to stand alone.

The purpose of a seminar series is to offer a health education experience alternative to a traditional series of classes that are interdependent and require regular attendance. A seminar series will attract participants who often choose not to participate because they are unable to commit to an entire six- or eight-week course due to personal or professional time commitments. Obviously, a traditional lifestyle health education course will be more effective in bringing about change, but a seminar series is not only better than nothing, it also provides a less threatening point of entry into the program for fence-sitters. Participants should be able to get "completion credit" for attending a defined portion of the series.

Theme Events

A *theme event* is any health promotion event that is tied to a holiday, anniversary, or theme, such as ethnic cuisines; exercise styles; or city, national, or global events. Examples include events associated with National Heart Month, New Year's Day, Columbus Day, or Earth Day.

The advantage of designing an activity based on known holidays is that often a certain amount of publicity in the popular media will reinforce your messages. Additionally, some organizations will offer free materials that are directly applicable to your event. This is, of course, especially true with health-related days such as the Great American Smokeout, which is actively supported by the American Lung Association and American Cancer Society.

How to Use This Book

These four promotional concepts will be seen throughout the following pages. While many of the ideas presented in this text are complete enough to implement with or without modification, the ideas can also serve as a springboard for your own innovative activities.

Be sure to make notes in the margins and white space provided to capture your thoughts when they occur. You are encouraged to modify, expand, and create your own health promotion ideas that work.

CHAPTER 3

Nutrition

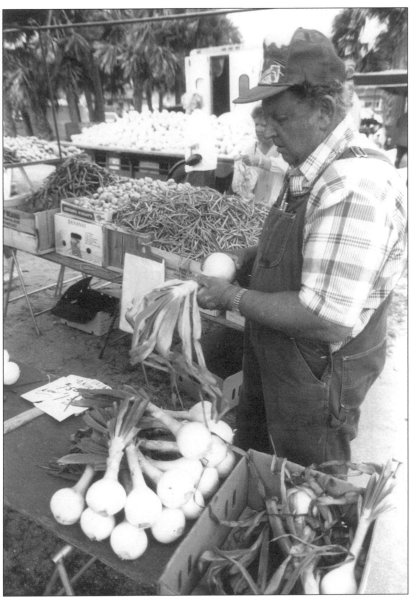

© Anthony Neste

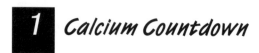 **1** *Calcium Countdown*

Monthly Minutes and seminar ideas support your female employees' health.

Use Monthly Minutes to increase awareness of the role of calcium in health and osteoporosis and especially as part of an overall strategy to support your women's-health objectives.

Starting Point

 Have lunchroom displays of over-the-counter calcium supplements and common foods with high calcium content.

 Offer samples of high-calcium foods along with handouts that include high-calcium recipes and information on osteoporosis.

 Conduct osteoporosis seminars that feature screening activities and prevention strategies.

 Hold nutritional seminars with an emphasis on the relationship between calcium intake and absorption, as well as strategies for increasing intake. Use log sheets to record calcium intake, and follow up with an individual or small-group analysis of results.

2 *Chinese New Year Celebration*

Celebrate the Chinese New Year with healthy Asian cooking.

Celebrate the Chinese New Year with a series of nutritional events designed around healthy Asian cooking. The Chinese New Year takes place on the second new moon after the Winter Solstice. It usually falls between January 21 and February 19, and the festivities last 15 days.

Starting Point

 Use this holiday as an opportunity to solicit a second round of health-related New Year's resolutions.

 Order customized fortune cookies with health-related fortunes of your choosing for distribution at appropriate events.

 Host a lunch called *Let's Take an Old-Fashioned Wok* featuring low-fat stir-fry cooking, samples, and recipes.

 Offer stir-fry cooking classes as a follow-up to the Monthly Minute.

 Offer related non-nutritional events during the celebration including martial arts classes, tai chi, and seminars on Eastern medicine like acupuncture and acupressure. Incorporate the 12 animals associated with your employees' birth years in your promotional strategies.

3 Employee Bakeoff

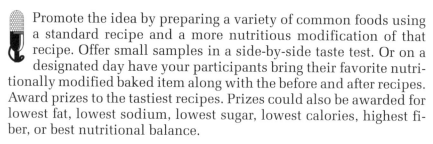

Raise the general awareness of nutrition with this activity that can reach all employee groups.

One method of increasing your employees' ability to make good nutritional decisions is to reinforce basic concepts of good nutrition and challenge their ability to modify their favorite recipes. An old-fashioned bakeoff can be used for this purpose.

Starting Point

 Offer classes or seminars on recipe modification and ingredient substitution. Include these concepts in your basic nutrition courses as well.

 Promote the idea by preparing a variety of common foods using a standard recipe and a more nutritious modification of that recipe. Offer small samples in a side-by-side taste test. Or on a designated day have your participants bring their favorite nutritionally modified baked item along with the before and after recipes. Award prizes to the tastiest recipes. Prizes could also be awarded for lowest fat, lowest sodium, lowest sugar, lowest calories, highest fiber, or best nutritional balance.

 Provide an ingredient substitution handout. Also promote the seminar nutritional modification contest.

 Hold a taste test in the cafeteria or other suitable location. Ask a number of highly visible members of management to be the taste testers.

Have a nutritionist evaluate the contest recipes for health-related factors and post or distribute the results.

 Publish the recipes in an employee cookbook and update it on a yearly basis. Identify "Flashback Food Fads" and "Oldies but Goodies" from the cookbook and sponsor a potluck dinner featuring these foods or have your cafeteria prepare them.

4 *Fall Harvest Festival*

*A vegetarian nutrition program that highlights the season's
fresh vegetables.*

In many areas of the country, the fall months offer a steady succession of fresh vegetables that are locally grown. Many of your employees will be reaping harvests of their own. Take advantage of this opportunity to promote some sound nutritional concepts. Here are some ideas your employees will "fall" for.

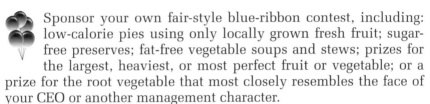

Starting Point

 Arrange for a farmer's market in your parking lot, inviting local growers to sell their freshest produce.

 Sponsor your own fair-style blue-ribbon contest, including: low-calorie pies using only locally grown fresh fruit; sugar-free preserves; fat-free vegetable soups and stews; prizes for the largest, heaviest, or most perfect fruit or vegetable; or a prize for the root vegetable that most closely resembles the face of your CEO or another management character.

Ask a nutrition consultant to judge the nutritional value of the recipes from the contests and post or distribute the results.

 Hold seminars on canning and preserving, including freeze drying and dehydrating fruits and vegetables.

5 *Have a Byte to Eat*

Promote your nutrition program with this high-tech activity.

Many employees are not aware of the nutritional content of their diets, even after attending nutritional education. They often focus on specific food items they are selecting rather than looking at their total diet over a period of time. They fool themselves into believing they are making good choices with occasional obvious decisions such as low-fat salad dressing. Give them a clearer picture of their choices with a computer diet analysis using one of the popular nutritional software programs.

Starting Point

A nutrition log can be handed out at a display table where employees sign up for nutritional analysis. Depending on staffing, equipment, and logistics, you can either complete the computer analysis and have the employee pick up the printout at the end of the lunch period, or have the participants complete the log and return it to your office for computer analysis.

Use the nutrition log to promote an upcoming nutrition education seminar. Have the participants drop off their logs at a work station that has been set up in the cafeteria. Participants pick up their results the following day or at the nutrition education seminar.

Tips for Success

- Select a software program and design an appropriate nutrition log for the period of time you wish to analyze. The most convenient choices are either for a 24-hour period or a single meal.
- Seminars offer the advantage of providing a personal contact with in-depth discussion where you can explain the results as well as give appropriate educational messages.

6 *Nuts Are Not What They're Cracked Up to Be!*

Use nuts to promote your nutrition courses.

Promote good nutrition with the often overlooked, but usually highly nutritious nut. Obtain a variety of nuts and go nuts! Some food distributors may donate these in exchange for some publicity.

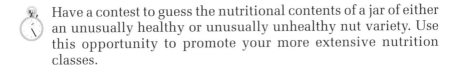

Starting Point

 Offer free samples of each type of nut and provide handouts on the nutritional content of each of the samples you are serving.

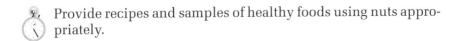 Have a contest to guess the nutritional contents of a jar of either an unusually healthy or unusually unhealthy nut variety. Use this opportunity to promote your more extensive nutrition classes.

Provide recipes and samples of healthy foods using nuts appropriately.

7 Restaurant Review Group

Rate the restaurants your employees frequent on your criteria for health.

If most employees go out for lunch, and in particular if your worksite is located near many restaurants, forming an employee restaurant review group may be an interesting addition to your nutrition activities. This activity can be used in conjunction with newsletters, bulletin boards, or handouts, or for a special publication.

Starting Point

Select a restaurant review team. Plan the entire event, including how you will communicate the results to the rest of the employees. Devise a schedule of outings, deadlines for newsletter articles, and publication deadlines. Schedule a training meeting with the group and a nutrition expert. Provide them with the basic knowledge, checklists, and review criteria needed to complete a review.

Distribute or post the group's review. Include criteria for low fat; low salt; low calories; high fiber; overall nutritional value; and of course variety, cost, service, ambiance, accomodations for nonsmokers, and the other usual restaurant review factors.

Tips for Success

- You can ask for volunteers, recruit individuals of your choice, or hold a drawing to select the review team.
- Be sure that the group is not only willing to commit to an extended (perhaps 12 months) assignment, but also is sincerely interested in contributing to your health promotion program.
- Having at least one individual with writing experience is useful.
- Schedule the first review session for the group and a nutrition consultant so the initial review can be conducted jointly.

8 *Salad Bar Buffet*

*Create a new tradition that supports your nutrition and
weight-control programs.*

Eating healthy and light is a challenge in America, but it is especially difficult at work if you are faced with limited options. One
way around this dilemma is to take charge of the options by organizing a regularly scheduled potluck buffet consisting of salad fixings.
This is especially well-received in smaller work groups with strong
social connections. It is also a good way to encourage interaction
among departments or individual employees, something that management generally likes to see.

Starting Points

 Use the salad bar buffet as a follow-up to a nutrition series. Post
a sign-up sheet with recommended ingredients to give the group
some guidance as to the quantities to bring. Encourage variety
and include some low-fat meats such as thinly sliced turkey.

 Organize themes, such as ethnic salads highlighting different
cultures (Mexican, Greek, or Asian, for example).

 Post the nutritional information of all the ingredients brought
to the buffet. Prepare a handout based on what participants sign
up to bring.

 Try kicking off the concept on St. Patrick's Day with *The Eating of the Green.*

Tips for Success

- Don't forget dressings (low-fat and low-calorie), paper plates,
  and utensils if needed. Request that everything be prepared
  (washed and sliced) before being brought to the buffet.
- Arrange for cold storage, either a refrigerator or several coolers.
- Solicit a volunteer leader to coordinate the event. Also remember to organize a cleanup crew.
- Agree on a designated time for the buffet to be served so everyone can share it.

9 *Summer Salad Celebration*

Schedule events to promote the first vegetables of the season as part of your nutritional program.

Throughout the late spring and early summer months, early seasonal fruits and vegetables are available in local markets freshly picked by local growers. Take advantage of the season by featuring these foods in your nutrition programming. Try some of these ideas:

Starting Points

 Offer gardening seminars in the late winter or early spring. Invite a local nursery or county or university extension specialist to speak on some appropriate topics such as soil testing and preparation, crop rotation, organic gardening principles, or Asian strip gardening.

 In conjunction with a gardening seminar series, organize group garden plots, charging a nominal fee for tilling and basic soil preparation if nearby land is available.

 Arrange for your food service to offer salads that feature unique combinations of available ingredients. Provide recipe handouts and nutritional information.

 Invite local growers to have a farmer's market in your parking lot. Or organize an employee farmer's market.

 Offer samples of low-fat and low-calorie salad dressings during the lunch hour.

 Host a brown-bag luncheon on salad and salad dressing preparation.

CHAPTER 4

Fitness

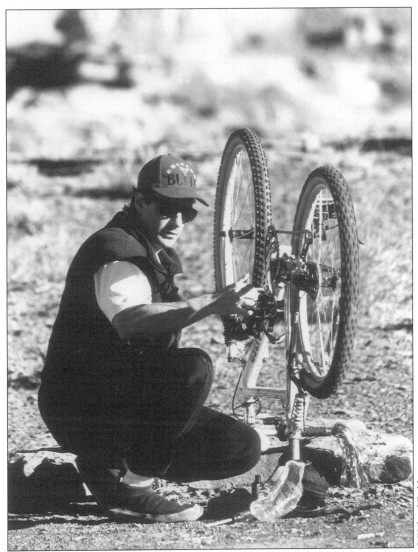

© Richard Etchberger

10 *Around the World in 80 Ways*

Follow the path created by Jules Verne on his trip around the world.

Take an exercise journey that offers an opportunity for anyone who exercises to participate. The total distance is approximately 25,000 miles and will require large numbers of participants in order to complete it within the suggested six to eight weeks.

Starting Point

 Use the basic principles of exercise journeys to plan the event. Chart the progress of the group effort on either a flat map of the world or a globe displayed in a prominent common area. Use an equatorial route, or duplicate the route described by Jules Verne in *Around the World in 80 Days*. Use group leaders from each group of exercisers to gather and report mileage.

Tips for Success

- Promote the event to begin on Jules Verne's birthday, which is February 8.
- Solicit the participation of all exercisers. For those who walk, swim, bike, run, ski, or skate, you can either use their actual mileage or use some common denominator to convert all activities into comparable numbers. The latter system will allow everyone to contribute equally no matter what their level of exercise. Time in aerobic exercise with walking as the common denominator is one such possibility. You can include stairclimbing, stationary rowing, biking, and treadmill walking to be converted into walking mileage.
- Read *Around the World in 80 Days* to pick up ideas for promotion and details that can be useful in organizing the event.
- Because the event is built on a literary theme, award gift certificates at a local bookstore to all participants who contribute during the entire event.

11 Celebrate Mardi Gras in New Orleans

Begin a swimming mileage event down the Mississippi and arrive in New Orleans in time for Fat Tuesday.

Here are some programs for swimmers that can transition right into a weight-control event. It can begin on the headwaters of the mighty Mississippi and pass through many scenic river towns along the way, ending in the Big Easy on Fat Tuesday. This event will require fairly large numbers of participants to be successful, but if you have an avid swimming population it can be a lot of fun.

Starting Point

 Beginning in Itasca State Park in north central Minnesota, the total distance to New Orleans is approximately 3,986 miles. The vertical drop (the difference between the elevation at the start of the river and the elevation at the mouth) is 1,679 feet. Post a map of the United States on your bulletin board to chart the progress of your participants. Write a day-by-day account of the trip with humorous anecdotes involving participants.

 Wear a Mardi Gras mask in your office on Fat Tuesday as you distribute incentive items. Be prepared to kick off a weight-control event at the end of the trip to take advantage of the visibility and uniqueness of Fat Tuesday.

Tips for Success

- Research some interesting facts from major stopping points along the route. Include general facts about the Mississippi. Consider Mark Twain connections in promoting the event—he is a rich source of quotations.
- If the total swimming mileage is accumulating too slow or too fast to make your destination on time, make daily adjustments in the current due to unexpected rainfall upstream, dams that were opened, or droughts. Use a range of 3 to 10 miles per hour in these adjustments.

12 Conquering Mount Everest and Other Lofty Pursuits

Convert your organization's stairwells into mountains for this popular exercise journey.

Exercise journeys up mountains are a popular way of adding physical activity to your employees' days by promoting use of the stairs in multilevel buildings or by promoting regular use of stairclimbers in your fitness facility. The premise is generally the same, but the details will vary with the target mountain and the history, geography, and culture of that locale.

Starting Point

 To prepare this journey, a few calculations are necessary. The total height of Mount Everest is 29,028 feet. The distance between floors in most office buildings is 13 feet. One way to set up this journey is to have participants climb upward 130 feet per day (10 floors) five days a week. "Trek teams" with four members each would need approximately 11 weeks to complete the event. Experience has shown that the teams may get competitive and will climb more than the estimated ten floors per day.

Trek teams should be formed with one person designated as the "Sherpa" to serve as team organizer and leader. On Mount Everest a Sherpa is a native who accompanies climbers, carrying much of their supplies. The Sherpa is very knowledgable about the mountain and climbers, and is a leader for the trek team. Team members report their climbing success each week to the Sherpa, who totals it and reports it to you. Alternatively, a drop box can be placed at the bottom of each stairwell with simple forms available for logging progress.

Tips for Success

- The timing of the event should coincide with some significant event. In the case of Mount Everest, you could use the anniversary of the first successful ascension by Sir Edmund Hillary in 1953; or the 1975 first ascent by a woman, Tabei Junko of Japan.
- Be warned that many participants will treat this exercise journey as a contest and they will actively pursue the fastest means to the top. Encourage your employees to add stairclimbing to their daily routines rather than trying to do a week's worth of climbing in one day.

- A chart depicting a mountain can be drawn on posterboard for tracking the progress of all teams. A vertical height scale should be included. Post this chart at the bottom or top of each stairwell.
- Update the chart weekly by placing numbered pins on the side of the mountain at the appropriate height.
- Track the progress of all teams on a computer spreadsheet so it is easy to compute totals and track progress. This will allow sorting by team name, total distance, etc. A printout of this spreadsheet can accompany the poster chart with weekly updates.

Other Target Mountains

- Mount Kilimanjaro in north Tanzania was first climbed by Hans Meyer and Ludwig Purtscheller in 1889. Kilimanjaro's height is 19,340 feet. It is the highest mountain in Africa.

- Mount Whitney in California was surveyed and measured by Josiah Dwight Whitney in 1864. This 14,494-foot peak was first climbed in 1864. It is the highest peak in the U.S. outside of Alaska.

- Mount McKinley is the highest mountain in North America at 20,320 feet. Discovered in 1794 by George Vancouver, it was first climbed by Hudson Stuck in 1913. You could link a walking exercise journey to the mountain then start a climbing journey. In remote mountain climbing you must often walk many miles before beginning the ascent. Mount McKinley is about 150 miles from Fairbanks, Alaska, in case you want to walk to it before climbing it.

- Mount Fuji is the highest mountain in Japan at 12,388 feet. It is usually climbed in July or August.

- Mount Washington in New Hampshire has a height of 6,288 feet. Time the activity with Presidents Day.

- The Nonnberg Abbey Mountainside in Austria, featured in *The Sound of Music,* is 14,100 feet high. Time the event with local Sommerfest activities and award participants "some of their favorite things."

Other lesser known mountains include:

- Mount Logan in the Yukon at 19,850 feet
- Aconcagua in the Andes of Argentina at 22,834 feet
- K2 in Kashmir at 28,250 feet
- The Matterhorn in Switzerland and Italy at 14,690 feet

13 *Iditasport*

Take a journey in March along the famed Iditarod Trail in Alaska.

Each year on the first Saturday in March, one of the world's most challenging endurance tests begins in Alaska. The Iditarod sled dog race covers 1,100 miles of rugged wilderness terrain under some of the most adverse conditions on the planet. It begins in Anchorage and ends in Nome. In Alaska, local agencies over the years have organized community events around the theme of Iditasport. Why reinvent the wheel? Take advantage of this concept and the publicity the Iditarod generates.

Starting Point

 Use the basic principles of exercise journeys to plan the event. Call your Iditarod an Iditawalk, Iditarun, Iditaswim, or Iditastairclimber. For planning purposes, the race is usually run in 10 days or so. (The most recent record, set in 1995, was 9 days, 2 hours, 42 minutes, and 19 seconds.) Or conduct multiple events simultaneously to involve exercisers from multiple areas of interest.

Tips for Success

- Information about the Iditarod is available from the Iditarod Trail Committee at 907-376-5155.
- Use a map of Alaska to chart the progress. Use the standard Iditarod checkpoints as intermediate goals.
- Use graphics portraying things like sled teams, igloos, and huskies.
- Your volunteer organizer for each team is designated as the "musher." Teams of exercisers consist of "huskies" with the participant contributing the most mileage during a given period of time or between checkpoints being designated "lead dog."

14 *Indianapolis 500*

Join your employees in the winner's circle as they walk, run, or bike 500 miles.

Every year as Memorial Day approaches, the media is full of information about the Indianapolis 500. This gives you an excellent opportunity to piggyback on this publicity.

Starting Point

Begin the event on Memorial Day, or preferably begin six to eight weeks before Memorial Day and target Memorial Day for a finish. Groups can be formed into racing teams with a leader who is designated as the driver.

The magic number for this program is 500. Five hundred miles of walking, running, swimming, or biking works well. Or 500 hours of other exercise like aerobics or strength training will also work. Team progress can be tracked in laps on an oval chart symbolizing the Indianapolis track. The distance around the Indy track is 2.5 miles.

The use of concepts such as tune-ups, maintenance, pit stops, pit crew, and other automotive or racing terms can be incorporated into seminar topics.

Tips for Success

- Use automobile-related incentive items such as small road atlases, car air fresheners, or coupons for discounts at a local oil change service.
- Teams should be named for automobiles.

15 │ *Walk a Mall in My Shoes*

Here is a low-intensity alternative for walkers, especially in very hot or very cold locations.

Many shopping malls have opened their doors to walkers, particularly during the winter, before or after their open hours. Here is an entry-level activity for very sedentary participants that takes advantage of the hospitality of shopping malls.

Starting Point

 Plan a walking route that covers an appropriate distance in a mall. Select stores at appropriate intervals as checkpoints and record some distinctive feature from their window display like sale prices, featured items, or unique displays. Formulate these facts into a scavenger hunt with a series of questions that participants must answer during the course of a walk.

Tips for Success

- Distribute a questionnaire with such questions as these: What is the price of the 25-foot tape measure displayed in the hardware store window? How many mannequins are in the window of the ABC women's clothing store? When does the sale at XYZ department store end?
- Design a route that takes about 15 to 20 minutes or a typical lunch period, as appropriate for your target audience. Keep in mind that many of the participants will be sedentary, so be conservative with the distance you expect them to travel.
- Encourage participants to walk the route in pairs and to discover answers to questions in the order you have indicated.
- Arrange for gift certificates valid in the mall as incentives to encourage shopping there. This is a nice gesture of appreciation for their cooperation.

16 *National Jogging Day*

Give your running and walking clubs a boost to get them through the winter.

National Jogging Day takes place in October and is an opportunity to either end the primary running season or, especially in northern regions, prepare and encourage participants to continue running through the difficult winter months.

Starting Point

 Organize a 10K/2K fun run. Consider including family members for team events (for example, father and son).

 Begin a journey based on running that culminates on either Thanksgiving or New Year's Day.

 Host a seminar on cold-weather running featuring both training methods and specialized clothing. Use the occasion to introduce running to interested nonrunners.

 Organize a series of events featuring motorized treadmills as an alternative to outdoor winter running. Promote active participation in your running club, especially for new members.

 Develop lists of locations such as local colleges and community sports facilities that are suitable for indoor running during the winter months. If possible, provide maps of the locations.

6O-Minute Triathlon

Give your employees a chance to train for this exciting challenge.

Triathlons became the event of choice for many elite athletes and fitness fanatics during the 1980s, and the event's popularity persists today. Competing in an actual triathlon, however, is often beyond the capabilities of the average person. A 60-minute triathlon can give participants some exercise goals to aim for while encouraging cross-training.

Starting Point

 The events to be used consist of either walking or running on a treadmill or track, biking on a stationary bike, and either swimming or rowing on a stationary rowing machine. Participants can begin training on one event at a time, working up to 20 minutes of continuous exercise on that event. They can then move to a combination of 20 minutes on one event with the addition of time on a second event, working toward a total of 40 minutes for the two events. They should rotate combinations of two events as they train. When they reach 20 minutes on each of two events, they should add the third event to their training session, building toward three 20-minute events.

In this event you can take two routes—set a goal of merely completing the entire 60 minutes of exercise, or set a date for the most total distance covered in the three events.

Tips for Success

- The triathlon is designed to be conducted in a fitness center environment. This can be either in an on-site facility or in a community fitness club.
- The 60-minute triathlon can be held either during the winter when outdoor exercise is more difficult in many parts of the country, or to coincide with a major triathlon such as the Ironman.
- When participants reach 20 minutes on each of two events, they should add the third event to their training session, building toward three 20-minute events. At this point participants should try to increase the distance they are able to cover in the 20-minute periods.

- You may set up separate competitions for various combinations of events (such as running, stationary bike, and swimming for participants with higher fitness levels) and equalize the resistance factors on the machines to create a level playing field. This will appeal to the employees with higher fitness levels and those who are most competitive. Participants with lower fitness levels can be rewarded for achieving personal goals.

18 *Summer Time and the Living Is Easy*

A fitness program with a Porgy and Bess *theme.*

Use themes from the musical *Porgy and Bess* to bring a low-key program to those slow summer months. Introduce employees to basic skills of lifetime sports so they can pursue a *Sporting Life.*

Starting Point

 Organize beginning lessons for lifetime sports such as archery, badminton, biking, in-line skating, swimming, racquetball, and tennis. Combine this activity with a community resource health fair to expose employees to all of the opportunities for lifetime sports in their area.

 Support lifetime sporting activities by cosponsoring leagues or clubs with local community recreation departments or the employee recreation club.

Tips for Success

- Modify the event to suit the needs of retirees if they are part of your eligible population.

19 *Spring Bike Tune-Up*

Kick off your bike club's session with informative tune-up sessions.

One of the obstacles to enjoyable biking is the hassle of keeping today's more complicated bicycles in perfect running order. A binding chain or derailer that jumps can be frustrating enough to keep fence-sitting bikers on their couch instead of their bike saddles.

Starting Point

 Invite a local bicycle repair person to present the seminar, which could be either lecture and demonstration or hands-on, depending on your physical space restrictions.

 Have an entire biking season planned for the club, including weekly rides, weekend tours, and/or a season-ending overnight ride. Designate a participant leader in advance to use the seminar as a promotion for a biking club.

Tips for Success

- Offer an incentive to participate, such as small sample-size cans of chain lube, a tire repair kit, or chances to win a riding garment.
- Since biking is such a good family activity, be sure to invite dependents.
- Use either a broken bicycle or bicycle wheel as a prop to draw attention to the preseminar promotion.
- Have a kickoff ride and sign-up strategy in place to be used during the seminar.
- Be prepared to keep the momentum going at season end with some stationary biking events.

20 *Spring Training*

*Join the boys of summer in preparation for your favorite
physical activity.*

In many work settings, the spring months offer an excellent opportunity to reach employees at a number of levels. First, some have been sedentary all winter and get the urge to begin some form of fitness activity in the spring. Second, some athletes, while generally in good shape, are switching sports and need some sport-specific conditioning. And third, there are those potential participants whose only fitness activity is participation in community-sponsored sports leagues such as softball, tennis, or golf. These people are in notoriously poor physical condition and tend to suffer soft-tissue injuries as a result of their weekend athlete behaviors.

Starting Point

 Time your event to coincide with either major league baseball's opening of spring training, or that of a local college or university. Use a spring camp format.

 Prepare handouts with sport-specific stretching guides.

 Prepare customized sport-specific strength workouts for use in your fitness center or with participants' private clubs, or prepare customized sport-specific calisthenics-based workouts for employees who do not have access to equipment.

 Offer single- or multiple-session introductory seminars on any or all of these topics to guide participants through the process of getting in shape. Bring in local high school or college coaches to conduct fundamental skills sessions for golf, softball, walking, running, and biking.

 Host an athletic training session to discuss first aid and home treatment for common sports injuries.

 Consider offering some public service education for nonfitness-related activities such as fishing or gardening.

21 Spring Wake-up Call

Get out of hibernation and get moving again!

Using the signs of spring as touchstones offers many opportunities to build on the concept of waking up after a winter hibernation. Help your employees re-energize after the long winter period.

Starting Point

 Play off the sleeping theme with a seminar on sleep including information on insomnia, differences among common mattress options, and health-related aspects of sleep.

 Focus on sedentary individuals who may have been "hibernating" their entire lives and offer programs with low-intensity fitness activities as well as training in sports fundamentals. For those regular exercisers who have merely slowed down over the winter, offer general fitness activities that begin at the beginning, like a running program that begins with walking.

 Offer seminars that promote the benefits of exercise in raising metabolic rates.

 Offer stretching classes that capitalize on the concept of yawning when waking up.

Tips for Success

- Use graphics involving bears, dens, and similar scenes on flyers and bulletin boards. You might even want to consider a Rip Van Winkle theme.
- Spring housekeeping can also be incorporated into the promotion.
- Nonparticipants and the very sedentary, who are often in the shadow of the fitness fanatics, will appreciate programming designed specifically for them.

22 *Swim the English Channel*

Have your fitness swimmers take on the challenge of the channel in this August exercise journey.

As low-impact aerobic activities gain popularity, it is important to offer promotional activities for those who participate in them. Here are some ideas for swimmers for the month of August, the month most channel swims take place, as well as a month that doesn't have many interesting events with which you can associate your program.

Starting Point

Use the basic principles of exercise journeys to plan the event. The distance across the channel is approximately 21 miles. The crossing takes place at the narrowest point beginning in Dover and ending in Calais. Set up teams of swimmers.

Tips for Success

- You can choose one of the following anniversaries for timing the event, or run it between these dates. The first successful crossing of the English Channel was done by Captain Matthew Webb on August 24 and 25 in 1875. His time was 21 hours and 45 minutes.
- The first woman to swim the channel was Gertrude Ederle, who did it on August 6, 1926, in 14 hours and 31 minutes.
- Another possible date for the event could be in conjunction with the Normandy Invasion in World War II, which is commemorated on June 6.
- Consider incentives with either a French or English theme for participants who complete the event, like a French toast breakfast at a local restaurant, English muffins, English breakfast tea, or French bread.

23 *Walktoberfest*

An old German tradition comes to health promotion.

Based on the traditional German Oktoberfest, develop a fall walking promotion around this concept (sans the beer and bratwurst). Walking should be a mainstay of any health promotion program and needs regular highlighting. Some of these ideas can help keep your walking programs going.

Starting Point

 Use your walking club to organize a Walktoberfest or use the event to organize a walking club. Have your cafeteria participate by serving healthy German-style lunches. Serve nonalcoholic beer and hire a band to play traditional German folk tunes during the event.

 Develop an exercise journey with an Oktoberfest theme.

 Offer seminars or demonstrations on speedwalking or powerwalking.

 Organize a family Volksmarch in the European tradition. Designate planned and measured walking routes within easy reach of your worksite. Or involve local community recreation departments for a more expanded event.

 Conduct a litter cleanup while walking over your designated walking routes.

 Consider repeating or continuing some of these activities during the winter months at local shopping malls or other available facilities with a new theme of *Walking in a Winter Wonderland, Walking in an Indoor Wonderland,* or *Walking in a Winter Indoorland.*

Tips for Success

- Contact local indoor shopping malls and gather relevant information on their walking routes. If they haven't yet developed public walking policies, plan to lobby to this end.

CHAPTER 5

Stress Management and Mental Health

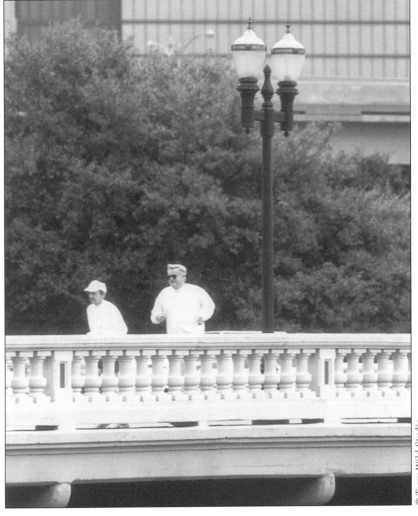

© Terry Wild Studio

24 *Cabin Fever Reliever*

*Break out of the long winter season with
stress management activities.*

Cabin fever is the generic term that describes the eagerness of people to get outside when they have been cooped up too long, generally over the winter months, and may have experienced mild depression. This is more a general condition in an individual's personal life rather than a work-related issue. However, cabin fever can adversely affect a person's productivity. This is an appropriate opportunity to work with your employee assistance program (EAP) or other company psychological services in preparing for this event.

Starting Point

 Offer seminars on such topics as Seasonal Affective Disorder, indoor air quality, humor, indoor winter activities, or the use of indoor plants in stress management.

25 *Don't Be a Crab*

Teach your employees about depression during July, the month of Cancer.

Here is an opportunity for a stress management Monthly Minute that is tied to an astrology theme. Plan this event in July, or more specifically from June 22 to July 22, the dates associated with the astrological sign of Cancer (the crab).

Starting Point

 Create stress management astrology readings and hand them out as part of a Monthly Minute (see Promotion #56, chapter 9).

 Hold an attitude adjustment seminar featuring humor and the role of positive attitudes in relationships, personal achievement, and mood.

 Use the astrology themes to promote any of your standard stress management activities.

26 Humorfest

A low-key stress reliever for hard times.

While this idea can be implemented at any time as a stress management activity, it is particularly appropriate when the workplace is going through difficult times. For example, if an organization is reducing its workforce, many health promotion activities that are typically fun and offer incentives are inappropriate. Employees in the midst of dramatic and threatening workplace changes will be offended by programming efforts that seem out of context and irrelevant. Try offering a humorfest for no reason other than relieving stress.

Starting Point

 Obtain videotapes or films of classic slapstick comedies like Laurel and Hardy, the Three Stooges, and the Marx Brothers. Modern comedies will be fine, too, but their length makes them less practical. Prepare and offer free air-popped popcorn or similar treats.

Tips for Success

- Reserve a large conference room where eating is permissible, or use a portion of the cafeteria that is suitable for the event. Show the films continuously during the lunch period.
- Advertise the event as a drop-in activity with no registration required.
- During these very difficult times, it is important to respect the needs of the employees and pay more attention to where they are currently rather than looking at their long-term needs. While they are in an extremely stressful environment and perhaps even in fear of losing their jobs, they probably are not well-served by smoking cessation, weight-control, or other more difficult behavioral change programs. Avoid pressure tactics for additional activity registrations and ride out the hard times with a sense of humor.

27 *Relaxation Room*

Give your employees a refuge from the craziness of the day.

One of the most insidious characteristics in many work settings is the lack of privacy, quiet, or even the availability of uninterrupted work time. Phones, meetings, machinery, noise, interruptions, and other normal activities can lead to a buildup of stress in many employees. Provide employees with an island of tranquillity by creating a relaxation room.

Starting Point

 Work with the person responsible for facilities decisions to locate a suitable space to set up a relaxation room. Possibilities include spaces like unused or underused closets or meeting rooms. Promote the use of the room by individuals or small groups at appropriate times to break the pattern of stress buildup during the workday.

Tips for Success

- As an alternative to dedicated space, try to block out times in conference rooms as available for relaxation only. This may be difficult in many organizations, but will certainly be a test of management support for your program.
- If you can arrange for a dedicated space, provide comfortable seating and low light.
- Arrange for the availability of a tape recorder either on a checkout basis or as a permanent fixture in the room. Provide an assortment of relaxation tapes, including structured progressive deep muscle relaxation, visualization scripts, nature sounds with or without music, and soft, relaxing music.
- This is an idea that may have sensitivity in some settings. It is possible that your management might fear the appearance of endorsing a religious belief associated with meditation, so be sure to get approval for this program. To avoid resistance from employees and management, try using the word *relaxation,* which sounds more secular than *meditation.*

28 *People Kneading People*

Introduce massage in a nonthreatening partner activity.

The benefits of massage as a form of relaxation are enjoyed by millions of people every day. However, not everyone can afford the time or money to take advantage of this wonderful therapy. For many people, a brief shoulder and neck massage can go a long way toward relieving their stress symptoms.

Starting Point

 Organize and promote a seminar to teach your employees basic, nonthreatening upper-body partner massage.

 Provide handouts with a structured 10-minute routine suitable for use between any two partners at the workplace.

 Promote the activity as a follow-up to stress management classes or as a stand-alone activity.

Tips for Success

- Target employees in jobs where upper-body tension is prevalent, such as those working for extended time periods on keyboards.
- Encourage continued participation during normal break times instead of snacking or smoking.
- Be sure to check out how appropriate this activity would be in your specific organization. Management or the participants themselves may have objections for a variety of reasons.

29 *Relax Fax*

Take advantage of technology to reach remote populations.

One of the most difficult challenges for health promotion professionals is delivering services to a dispersed population such as field sales or other branch offices, especially when employee populations are too small to justify great expenditures of time. In order to work with these groups, the use of technology is an essential strategy.

Starting Point

Plan a series of one-page faxes on stress management. The nature of these faxes will vary depending on whether they will be used as posters or handouts. Establish a working relationship with one contact person in each target office. This person will receive and copy, distribute, or post the fax.

Look for other opportunities to use the fax machine, such as weight-management weekly hints; two-way communication for group contests or exercise journeys; sharing of nutritional information or recipes; or conducting surveys for program planning. Also, look for related communications opportunities such as voice mail, e-mail, and electronic bulletin boards.

Tips for Success

- Develop a group mailing list for "batching" faxes. Since you may be transmitting for an extended time period, plan on using a delayed transmission feature if you have it. This will allow you to transmit during the night or at other times that are less likely to conflict with others' needs.
- Content ideas for the faxes could include general educational information about stress; strategies for stress reduction or management; site-specific program- or community-based stress management opportunities; or registration forms for enrolling in self-study stress management activities if they are available.

Sigmund Freud's Birthday Party

A light-hearted way to promote your EAP.

EAP and health promotion share similar organizational goals and are a natural complement to each other. EAP, however, often suffers relatively low utilization due to its position in the employee population. It can carry some stigma, and, in order to maximize its potential, requires promotion. Here is an opportunity to integrate your services with those offered by the EAP. Consider holding a reintroduction of the EAP and its capabilities on the birthday of Sigmund Freud, the founder of psychoanalysis. The date is May 6, 1856. Be sensitive to the nature of many employees' problems in designing this event.

Starting Point

 Promote the nonclinical aspects of an EAP with a money management seminar, a speaker on Alzheimer's disease (offered as an elder care service), a session on selecting child care providers, a workshop on managing change, a Meyers-Briggs personality type workshop, or a speaker addressing relationships.

 Organize an on-site Alcoholics Anonymous (AA) group.

Tips for Success

- Meyers-Briggs personality type workshops are available through organizational development consultants and often within the human resources department in large organizations.
- Be sure to work with your EAP counselors or vendor in AA groups. There may be contractual concerns or turf issues that need to be resolved before proceeding.

31 *S.O.S. (Stamp Out Stress)*

A perfect theme for May Day.

Another opportune time to focus on stress is on the first day of May, known worldwide as May Day. Paradoxically, *mayday* is also the universal distress signal. Focus an entire month on stress management.

Starting Point

 Sponsor appropriate Monthly Minutes such as stress logs or stress dots. Stress dots, often called biodots, are small appliqués that change color with temperature change. When placed on the hand they can detect stress-induced changes in skin temperature. Stress logs are distributed with guidelines for use. Have participants log their stressful symptoms in relation to events that occur during the day. Stress dots handed out at the entrance to the building on Mondays and Fridays show the difference that attitude can make.

 Conduct a biofeedback demonstration to illustrate an individual's ability to affect sympathetic nervous functions. Or offer a seminar series featuring single sessions that focus on stress reduction techniques—deep muscle relaxation, visualization, music, and exercise.

Conduct a seminar on the role of pets in stress reduction.

 Host introductory yoga classes with an opportunity for an ongoing activity.

Tips for Success

- Be sure to include speakers from the EAP who can promote the services they offer.
- Of course, don't forget to kick off your standard stress management class.

32 *Stress Cards*

Monthly Minutes to promote your stress management program.

Here's a very inexpensive Monthly Minute that is highly visible and allows for individual interaction with participants. The only materials needed are a biofeedback stress card, which is available from a wide variety of sources, including Teraco Products (see appendix), and your handouts.

Starting Point

Offer an informal stress check. During the check, inform the participant about the activity you wish to promote. Create a two-sided handout with "Ten Things You Can Do to Reduce Stress This Week" on one side and information about and a registration form for the event on the other side.

Tips for Success

- Plan the event for lunch and/or break periods in a lunchroom setting.
- Promote the event with table tents so that anyone sitting at a table will see the promotion.
- Choose a highly visible location.
- Have participants grasp the card according to the instructions. Even though the instructions indicate holding about 10 seconds, ask participants to hold it for 30 to 45 seconds. This will give you a captive audience for that time period.
- Build in a tear-off form for a chance in a raffle as part of the handout.

33 *Stress Management for Special Populations*

Revive interest in stress management classes.

One of the unique characteristics of stress is that it is a very personal issue. Many people rightfully believe they are among the most stressed individuals in the workforce. They feel that their situations are unique and for this reason, generic stress management classes are fine for the general population but not for them. Try using this information to create a more successful stress management program with the following tactics.

Starting Point

 Promote the class specifically to the target audience; for example, *Secretarial Stress* or *Coping on the 16th Floor.* Only allow members of the target audience to attend. Select an instructor who has knowledge about or experience working with the target population.

Tips for Success

- Analyze the demographics of your workforce, health risk assessment data, participant surveys, or marketing data and look for concentrations that would be likely candidates for stress management. One of the most common factors around which the need for specialization will cluster is job type—for example, clerical, sales, management, and so on.
- This customization technique can be applied to many activities and will usually result in better participation and more successful results.
- Redesign the content of a standard stress management class to match the needs of the target population. Consider
  — length of class sessions—nonexempt employees may need shorter blocks of time due to work schedules;
  — time and location of the class;
  — examples used within the class to illustrate points; and
  — strategies and interventions appropriate to socioeconomic status.

34 *Untie the Stress*

Introduce casual dress at the workplace as one tool to reduce stress.

Casual dress-down days are becoming more common throughout the business world. If your workplace hasn't adopted this convention, consider hosting an *Untie the Stress* day to introduce the concept with a few easy steps.

Starting Point

 Obtain the blessing of management to implement the project. Combine this day with other stress management activities to highlight the purpose of the event.

Tips for Success

- Give employees plenty of advance notice as well as a reminder when they leave work the day before the event.
- Request sensible "business casual" clothing be worn for the day. Some rules may have to be established depending on the culture, norms, and type of business.

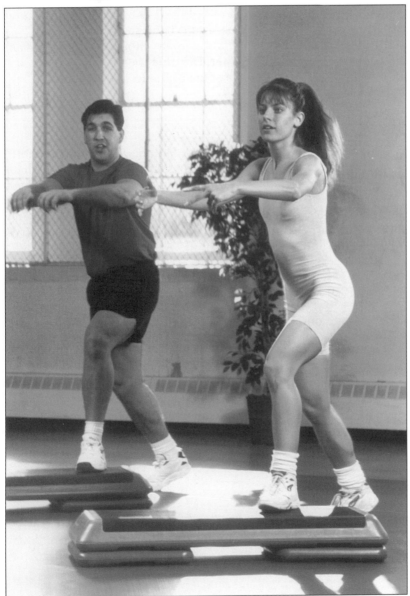

CHAPTER 6

Weight Control

© Terry Wild Studio

35 *Are You Afraid of Your Shadow?*

A six-week weight-control event just in time for spring.

Legend indicates that on February 2, across the country in cold climates, the groundhogs come out of their dens after a long winter hibernation. If a groundhog looks around and sees its shadow, it gets scared and goes back into hibernation for six more weeks. This event predicts six more weeks of winter. Use this theme to kick off a six-week weight-control event with some of the following ideas.

Starting Point

 Announce the event with a *Name That Shadow* contest. Photograph willing executives' shadows in profile. Post the shadows on a bulletin board and have employees match the shadows with the correct names. The core activities will of course be similar to many other weight-control activities with weigh-ins, support information, and concurrent weight-control classes. This event is simply a fun way to kick it off.

Tips for Success

- Incorporate one or more spring fitness ideas into the program.
- Use this as a kickoff for *Spring Meltdown* (Promotion #39).

36 Budget Your Calories

A weight-control program built around the annual budget planning cycle.

Every year most organizations go through the annual budget cycle. This is a generally dreaded process that involves creating a budget based on your proposed plan for the coming year, then submitting it only to have it returned with a request to cut your proposal by some percentage, then resubmitting it. The process will usually have high visibility within the organization and is a natural time to piggyback a health promotion program. Try coordinating a weight-control program using this financial theme with some of these ideas.

Starting Point

 Develop daily, weekly, and monthly calorie logs based on a financial spreadsheet. Include income or revenue (food intake) and expense or output (exercise) columns. Include a special column for tracking calories derived from fat. Set budget goals that support weight-control goals. Time the event with current organizational timing of budget submission or monthly forecast submissions. Extend the program at least through the entire budget planning cycle.

Tips for Success

- Provide participants with information to assist with calorie tracking for both diet and exercise with the following:
  — Seminars or classes
  — Convenient handouts and charts
  — Nutritional labeling of all items offered in vending machines or the cafeteria
  — Copies of menus of popular local restaurants with calorie estimates
- Incorporate financial terminology into your communications and promotions like deficits, shortfall, debit, credit, saving, planning, budgeting, and budget cutting.

37 Hollywood Stars

A weight-control activity for your celebrity employees.

Weight-control contests are a popular activity in most programs. Here's one theme that can be implemented easily and inexpensively.

Starting Point

 Each participant chooses a code name (the name of a celebrity). Have all participants weigh in with you at the beginning of the contest. Create a chart on which to post all of the participant's names, ensuring enough columns to record a weight once a week for six to eight weeks. For the first week, enter a weight of zero for all participants. Have participants weigh in each week and record the difference from the starting point on the chart. At the conclusion of the event, give participants appropriate feedback and congratulatory messages for the motivation and effort shown both by those who were successful in achieving their goals and those who weren't.

Tips for Success

- Schedule this activity to coincide with the Academy Awards. Set up a pool with participants guessing who will win in the most common award categories such as best film, best director, or others that seem appropriate. Provide modest prizes for the winners of the pool.
- Each participant should set personal goals that are appropriate.
- Each week participants should be given some type of support material such as a "Hint of the Week."
- Rather than recording actual weight, record weight in relation to an individual's starting point. For example, if Jane Doe loses 2 pounds, record a -2 for that week. Each week the recorded weight will always be in relation to the first week's starting point of zero.
- Include a nominal incentive item and promotional material for more formal weight-management programs that have been scheduled to follow the activity.

38 *Pinch an Inch*

Promote your weight-control program with this simple test.

Every weight-control effort should include some aspect of body composition education, either establishing baselines or at least introducing the concept to participants. Here is a simple Monthly Minute based on skinfold measurements.

Starting Point

Obtain skinfold calipers. Use a one-site pinch test that tests the back of the arm on the triceps. Give employees the test and a brief verbal pitch for your seminar. Prepare handouts that contain basic information on body composition, registration information for your future event, and space to indicate the results of a participant's test.

Use the skinfold test to promote either a seminar on body composition or a weight-control event. Topics can include:

- Multisite pinch test
- Electrical impedance test
- Infrared test
- Body composition versus ideal body weight
- Improving body composition
- Upcoming weight-control or fitness activities

Tips for Success

- For the purpose of this activity, even the most inexpensive calipers will do. While this is not the most accurate estimate of body composition, it serves as a point of discussion that will hopefully lead participants to a more accurate test at your seminar. Consider using Human Kinetics's Practical Body Composition Kit for this activity. It is available by calling 1-800-747-4457 or visiting the Human Kinetics web site at **http://www.humankinetics.com/**.

39 *Spring Meltdown*

Get in sync with the seasons and begin to melt your pounds away.

In most areas of the country that receive snowfall and have rivers and lakes that freeze over, the spring thaw is an annual event that is welcomed by all. At this time of the year, many people are looking forward to warmer weather when they will be able to wear shorts, bathing suits, and other more revealing clothing. This phenomenon can be used as a platform for another weight-control event, *Spring Meltdown.* Try incorporating some of these ideas with your own.

Starting Point

 Develop a weight-control event. Organize a group weigh-in to establish the baseline, which can be represented as the snow-pack. Chart the group's progress through these visuals after a weekly group weigh-in.

 Host a spring "runoff" (including walkers) to kick off some spring fitness support activities or incorporate spring skiing or related themes in your planning.

Tips for Success

- Piggyback this event with another like *Are You Afraid of Your Shadow?* (Promotion #35).
- Create visuals using charts depicting snow melting from a mountain, or a layer of snowpack that will get thinner as the event progresses. (See *We're All in It Together,* Promotion #41).
- Rent a snowcone machine and offer free snowcones in the cafeteria at the conclusion of the event to draw attention to it and to your next related event.

40 *Weighting for the New Year*

Begin a weight-control program that will carry employees through the holidays.

The holiday season is a difficult time for anyone concerned about weight. Beginning with the Thanksgiving meal, the feast continues through holiday office parties and numerous other social occasions involving eating and drinking. We have way too many opportunities to eat during the holidays! The average person stands a good chance of gaining several pounds during this vulnerable time.

Starting Point

 After appropriate promotion, have participants weigh in with you just before Thanksgiving. Have everyone set a goal of zero weight gain for the duration of the event. During a period where weight gain is the norm, maintenance can be viewed as progress. Record their weight confidentially. At remote locations, have employees weigh in with a partner and submit the information to you. Have a mid-December progress report weigh-in to spot individuals who have had problems during the Thanksgiving and post-Thanksgiving period. Hold a final weigh-in after employees return to work after New Year's Day.

 Offer weekly written support information including traditional weight-control hints, low-calorie and low-fat Thanksgiving recipes, eating at two or more family gatherings, sensible holiday drinking, and low-calorie party recipes.

Tips for Success

- Offer backsliders special attention such as brown-bag luncheons; weekly or daily weigh-ins; and personal words of encouragement by e-mail, voice mail, or phone call.
- Provide incentive items for everyone who met their goals as well as appropriate items that recognize the effort of those who did not.

41 *We're All in It Together*

A group weight-control activity with a twist.

This activity is best done in an environment where a large freight scale is available. It is useful in any weight-control activity involving teams or departments.

Starting Point

 At a predetermined time like break or lunch, gather teams at the freight scale. Have one team or department step on the scale together. Competing teams or departments witness the weight of the entire group. Have the group do a group hug on the scale. Repeat with all teams.

Tips for Success

- This event is one way of incorporating everyone in a group in the event. Even those who don't need to lose weight can support those who do by maintaining their weight.
- Participants who could stand to lose a few pounds but are not sufficiently motivated to do it on their own can contribute to the group effort.
- The fact that the weigh-in is witnessed by other teams adds to the sense of commitment to the group goal.
- Be careful to structure the event to foster healthy weight control rather than a competitive frenzy that could lead to rapid or extensive weight loss by highly competitive individuals.

CHAPTER 7

Smoking Cessation and Cancer Prevention

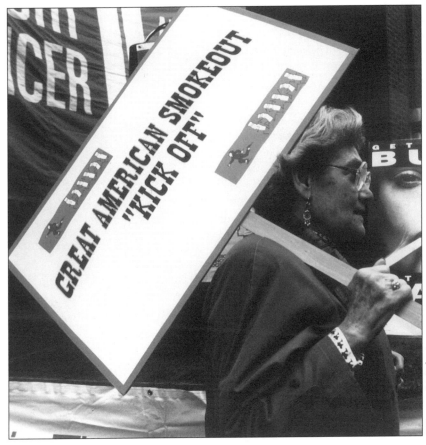

© Frances M. Roberts

42 Cancer Countdown

Recognize National Cancer Month with a series of events.

Recognize National Cancer Month with a series of events supporting cancer-reducing health behaviors. Cancer research is revealing new information at a steady pace. Keep your participants current with a series of brown-bag luncheons on cancer-related topics. Here are a few seminar ideas to consider.

Starting Point

 From the Rainforests to You—A status report on the ozone layer and skin cancer, or the role of exotic plants in medical research.

 Tales from the Cabbage Patch—What cancer prevention can you expect from dietary interventions?

 From Mammography to Menopause—What can you do to prevent breast cancer?

 Testicular Self-Examination and Prostate Examination—Simple prevention techniques for men.

43 *Celebrate Independence From Smoking*

A Declaration of Independence from unhealthy lifestyles and a midyear look at personal health goals.

The Fourth of July is the anniversary of the signing of the Declaration of Independence. This presents another opportunity for promoting gaining independence from any unhealthy habit. Here are some ideas that relate to smoking.

Starting Point

 Re-enact the signing of the Declaration of Independence, using management personnel in signing the document. Draft a one-page "Declaration" that is modeled after the original but is related to smoking. Post and circulate the signed document. The period of independence can vary— just the day, the entire holiday weekend, or a permanent commitment. Have everyone willing to attempt quitting also sign the document.

Tips for Success

- Incorporate a graphic of George Washington's wooden teeth, clearly stained brown, in printed materials that illustrate reasons to quit smoking other than those associated with health.
- Incorporate a fireworks theme—*Do a Bang-Up Job With Your Health.*

44 *Fry Now, Pay Later*

Prevent skin cancer through sensible outdoor exposure to the sun.

Skin cancer is one of the most preventable cancers. Try this Monthly Minute to raise awareness and promote your informational seminar.

Starting Point

 Hand out sample-sized bottles of sunscreen, inexpensive sunglasses, or sunscreen lip balm to attract participants. Include an educational handout or seminar notice.

 Set up a series of seminars with invited speakers to talk on the subject of skin cancer. Topics might include:

- A self-test to determine one's risk
- An explanation of proper sunscreen use
- UV rays and eyewear
- Early detection of skin cancer
- The U.S. Weather Service's UV Index
- Sport-specific hints for skiing, fishing, boating, and other high-risk activities

45 *Great American Smokeout*

Don't miss out on this national event, but be prepared to give it a new look with new ideas!

The next logical time for smoking cessation activities is in November during the Great American Smokeout. The American Cancer Society offers excellent supporting materials for this national event. Here are a few other ideas that relate to this core activity.

Starting Point

Offer smoked turkey sandwiches in the cafeteria as a featured entree during a *Going Cold Turkey* promotional event. Give coupons offering discounts toward the registration fees for smoking cessation classes as part of an incentive program.

Conduct a *Flick a Butt* contest for willing participants outside the building as they enter. Make this part of your *No Ifs, Ands, or Butts* program. Draw an appropriate target on the ground and have employees flick their last cigarette butt of the day for accuracy or distance. Give them additional chances in a drawing for a prize for the best accuracy. Give incentives and support materials to all participants.

Hold a *Guess the Number of Butts in the Jar* contest with the following steps. Collect 24 hours' worth of butts from building ashtrays (do it for a week in small facilities). Place them in a closed jar to display in the lobby or cafeteria. Have participants guess the number of butts in the jar for chances in a drawing or other prize system. Offer hints such as the amount of money spent on smoking those cigarettes, or the amount of government subsidy spent to grow them. Alongside the jar place another smaller container with a simulated amount of tar associated with the cigarettes. Use roofing tar or a similar substance.

Conduct a *Dare to Compare* event. Arrange for breath testing of either carbon monoxide or lung capacity. Place a piece of posterboard behind the activity table. On it, draw a vertical line down the center with a scale that is associated with the probable test results like carbon monoxide (CO) in parts per million (PPM). Offer your usual incentives to everyone who takes a test. As each person tests, place a small adhesive colored dot on the chart. On one side of the line, use red dots for smokers. On the other side, use blue dots for nonsmokers. As the day progresses, the red dots will cluster at higher CO levels or lower lung capacity levels than the blue dots. It will graphically illustrate some direct effects of smoking on a person's lungs.

46 *New Year's Resolutions*

A theme that capitalizes on traditional New Year's resolutions.

The first opportunity of the year is New Year's Day. Many people are motivated to make a commitment to one or more changes through resolutions. Most smokers are well-informed about the health risks associated with smoking. The continuing challenge is to draw them into appropriate interventions that will be successful in helping them quit.

Starting Point

 Encourage participants to work on their most serious risk (which for smokers will most likely be smoking). Emphasize focusing on only one area at a time to keep the process from overwhelming them. Strengthen their commitment to change by asking them to share their resolution either publicly or at least with a person significant to them.

Tips for Success

- Provide supporting activities specific to smoking cessation.
- Provide activities that support the commitment to change.
- Be prepared for ongoing support activities to reduce recidivism.

47 *Smoking Cessation Readiness Classes*

Ease your smokers into behavior change with this program.

Many participants find the prospect of quitting smoking very threatening and even frightening. For this reason they aren't willing to consider making the attempt to quit. Yet we know that when they are ready, they will quit if the proper circumstances prevail at the time of the decision. Many employees attend smoking cessation program activities but don't quit while in the activity. They often consider themselves as having failed in the attempt. Some of them will go on to successfully quit later, on their own or in a second attempt in a program. Try drawing in these reluctant smokers by lowering the pain threshold with smoking cessation readiness classes during which they will not be asked to quit.

Starting Point

 Reorganize the content of your smoking cessation classes by eliminating the quit day. Emphasize tapering and the use of lower-nicotine cigarettes. Use the psychological principle of "shaping behavior" using small rewards to reinforce the small steps that move toward the desired final behavior of quitting smoking.

Tips for Success

- Invite your previous dropouts to participate.
- Choose the most compassionate instructor that you can find to teach the classes.

48 *Operation Clean Sweep*

A second opportunity to work with your smokers.

The next opportunity for change is any time in the spring, using a spring housecleaning theme. Here are some possibilities.

Starting Point

 If your organization hasn't implemented a clean air policy, this is a good time to do so and in the process clean the house. Use housecleaning tools in the graphics for your bulletin boards and flyers.

 A variation on the theme is *Operation Clean Sweep,* using concepts built around chimney sweeping. Make analogies between chimney sweeping and the natural cleansing process that takes place after one quits smoking. Provide information handouts and supporting materials to help participants quit.

CHAPTER 8

Work and Family

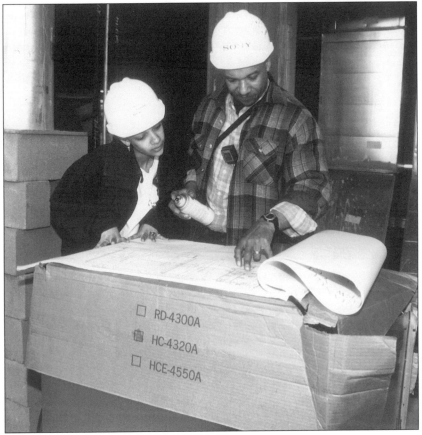

© Frances M. Roberts

49 *Family Health Care Fair*

Bring your community's child care providers to your parents to plan for the summer.

Family care issues are emerging as one of the most important areas affecting employees' productivity and quality of life. The economic necessities of the decade have made dual-income families the norm and achieving a balanced life a challenge. Here is an idea that can help parents cope with decisions about summer child care activities.

Starting Point

Host an event built around a health fair format. Design it specifically to address child care issues. Invite local care providers to display in booths or tables.

Tips for Success

- Remember to invite a variety of child care providers including day care referral agencies, summer day camps, summer specialty camps like computer camp or basketball camp, YMCA/YWCA, local school district summer school, nanny services, and the local park district.
- Host a temporary on-site day care service during the event to allow parents to experience the fair freely.

50 Father's Day

Father's Day offers an opportunity for a different look at parenting issues.

Awareness of the father's role in parenting has increased greatly in recent years. However, awareness certainly could be improved. You can increase awareness of the importance of the role of the father in child development and provide instruction in techniques and activities that your participants will find useful. Consider trying a seminar series with some of the following topics.

Starting Point

 Offer an early child care skills seminar using a pediatrics nurse to teach men about correctly bathing infants, diapering and cleaning up, food preparation and feeding, burping and hiccups, and properly dressing children for a variety of weather conditions.

 Conduct a seminar on the correct use of child restraint seats in automobiles. Include information about the selection and use of other child carriers like back carriers and front carriers.

 Plan a series of child health seminars covering topics like fevers and taking an infant's temperature, childhood diseases, immunizations and recordkeeping, regular checkups, medication dos and don'ts, and emergency care.

 Hold a seminar on early child development including information on the normal stages of child development, assisting with development (for example, helping a child learn to walk), identifying child development problems, and reading to your child.

Tips for Success

- Give a free copy of a popular child care book to the first ten attendees.
- Provide handouts after the seminars on where to get additional information and assistance. Also provide a summary of the seminar to participants.

Homecoming

An autumn work and family theme to help employees achieve balance in their lives.

For many couples, dual incomes have become a necessity for economic survival. These couples often find that the demands of their careers prevent them from balancing their work with their personal lives. Try a homecoming theme to bring them back to a more centered existence. Here are some ideas.

Starting Point

 Develop a seminar series. Discuss the central issue with your EAP representative to get a better idea of the problems your employees might be facing. Schedule seminar topics that relate to the problem, such as:

- Balancing your life
- Child care options in your community
- Effective interpersonal communications
- Communication differences between men and women
- Body language
- Time management in your personal life
- Quality time versus quantity time
- On-the-job assertiveness training
- How to say no

Tips for Success

- The best time for these activities is in the fall, especially if your town has a college football team or even an active high school football program.
- Time the seminar to coincide with the most visible local homecoming game. Adapt your local team name, mascot, and colors to your posters, flyers, and newsletter.
- Consider having follow-up classes of a more in-depth nature on the topics that appear to be most popular or most useful to your employees.
- Use the EAP as a resource to locate appropriate speakers. Providing speakers on EAP-related topics may even be part of their job description. This gives you an opportunity to integrate services while economizing on program costs.

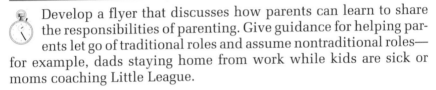

52 *Balancing the Scales of Your Life*

An activity to focus on bringing more balance into your participants' lives.

The astrological sign of Libra is represented by scales. The dates associated with Libra are from September 23 to October 23. This is a great time to promote personal balance.

Achieving a healthier balance in one's life can significantly contribute to improved mental and physical health and an overall sense of well-being. Promoting this well-being is a critical part of working with the whole person in your health promotion efforts. Parents need skills that allow them to fully participate in parenting while doing a better job of taking care of themselves. Here are some ideas that can help your participants move toward balance in their lives.

Starting Point

Develop a flyer that discusses how parents can learn to share the responsibilities of parenting. Give guidance for helping parents let go of traditional roles and assume nontraditional roles—for example, dads staying home from work while kids are sick or moms coaching Little League.

Plan a series of seminars on managing your family time. Include such topics as planning for personal time alone, planning for time with your partner, and planning time for one-on-one interaction with individual children, including time to play with your children and for your own recreation.

Conduct a seminar on work-related issues like putting work in perspective, time management at work, handling overtime, career management, interpersonal conflict at work, dealing with authority, and assertiveness.

Tips for Success

- Be sure to use your EAP as a resource in planning and delivering some of these activities.

53   *Mother's Day*

*Reintroduce some mothering activities to improve
participants' parenting.*

Consider promoting age-appropriate activities that might be categorized under the heading of "mothering"—practical and nurturing skills that improve the quality of family life and especially impact children. Include traditional mothering activities as well as nontraditional ones. Offer activities that are appropriate for and appeal to all members of the family. This may be particularly useful if your population is either in a lower socioeconomic group or has a large number of single-parent families.

Starting Point

Teach participants the basics of storytelling, including oral family history, fables, and fairy tales. Include information about traditional mothering activities like cooking, mending clothing, laundry (correctly operating machines), housecleaning, caring for personal belongings, basic home repair (unclogging toilets, changing fuses), automobile maintenance (changing the oil), and basic financial matters (writing a check, how credit cards work).

54   *Take Good Care of Your Womb Mate*

Celebrate Mother's Day with prenatal education.

Prenatal health care can be one of the most significant factors in reducing the risks of difficult pregnancies and deliveries, low-birthweight babies, and other complications. These problems can be a major health care expense for both organizations and parents. Bring attention to this issue with some of these ideas.

Starting Point

 Kick off your activities on the Monday following Labor Day. Organize a seminar series including some of the following topics:

- General prenatal nutrition information
- Nontraditional alternatives to prenatal care like herbs, vitamins, and yoga
- The effects of alcohol, caffeine, and tobacco use during pregnancy
- Exercise guidelines during pregnancy
- Losing weight following delivery
- Alternative delivery options like midwives or doulas
- Involving your partner in pregnancy and birth
- Planning for child care after the delivery
- Appropriate and extraordinary medical testing
- Weight-gain and weight-control guidelines
- Mental health issues common during and after pregnancy
- Risks associated with pregnancy at various stages
- Use of prescription and over-the-counter drugs

Feature a brief written test to determine whether your female employees who are either pregnant or planning on having children are in high-risk categories. This information is available from the March of Dimes.

Develop some of the seminar topics into a written format, including appropriate pamphlets available from the March of Dimes, your local HMO, or hospitals. Assemble them into packages that can be picked up or sent to remote locations.

CHAPTER 9

Holidays and Seasons

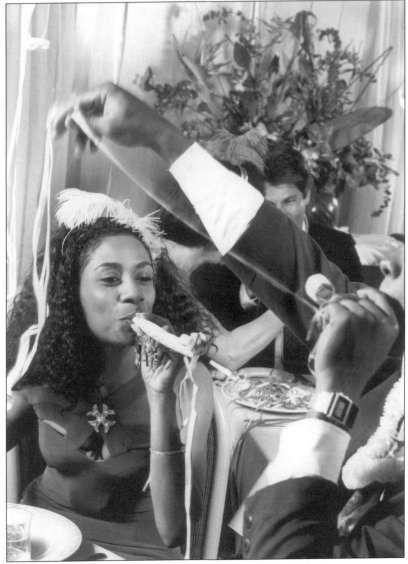

© Photo Network/Tom McCarthy

55 *Allergy Alert*

Just in time for summer, bring your employees up-to-date with the latest information on this annual nuisance.

Allergies of all types can not only make a person uncomfortable, but can actually prevent some from pursuing an active lifestyle. While fall and spring are particularly troublesome, and most appropriate for programming, the window of opportunity can be spread out to accommodate your schedule. Here are some topics for a seminar series.

Starting Point

 Develop a seminar series. Use some of the following topics: spring allergies, fall allergies, molds, animal allergies, food allergies, exercise-induced asthma, antihistamines, decongestants, inhalers and other allergy remedies, and allergies and asthma.

56 *Astrology Themes*

Help your employees determine their own healthy futures with these ideas.

The signs of the zodiac can be a source of ideas for promoting a variety of activities. You may not be able to devise a clever activity for every sign of the zodiac, but all signs can be incorporated into health-related readings. Here is a starter list of astrology-related ideas.

Starting Point

 Aquarius the Water Bearer (January 20 to February 18)—Start a water exercise program, or distribute information about the role of water in nutrition and health.

 Pisces the Fish (February 19 to March 20)—Pass out information on the role of fish in a nutritional diet. Hand out recipes and material about proper handling of fish and seafood.

 Gemini the Twins (May 21 to June 21)—Invite a speaker to discuss relationship-related activities with your employees. These activites should include primary relationships, family relationships, friendships, and work-related relationship topics.

 Cancer the Crab (June 22 to July 22)—Prepare cancer awareness and prevention or stress management materials to distribute to your employees.

 Leo the Lion (July 23 to August 22)—Conduct a mini-training course on assertiveness.

 Libra the Scales (September 23 to October 23)—Promote balance in your employees' lives by using any of the ideas listed in chapters 3, 4, or 6 to develop a weight-control and nutrition program.

 Scorpio the Scorpion (October 24 to November 21)—Prepare materials about poison control in the home.

Another option is to fabricate health-related astrology readings and promote involvement in an upcoming program. Other similar encouraging readings can be created to support your efforts. For example, for any given sign the readings could be: "You will enjoy success in physical endeavors. This is a good time for goal setting and new beginnings" or "Group activities can benefit you at this time. Look for support from your colleagues" or "Your personal power will increase in the near future. Pursue new directions physically."

57 *Back to School*

A program to educate your employees on basic back care and injury prevention techniques.

Acute back injuries and chronic back pain continue to be significant productivity and health-care claims problems for many companies. You can make a significant contribution to solving your organization's problems in this area with this fall theme. Here are some suggested activities.

Starting Point

 Develop back care classes cosponsored with your safety or occupational health departments. Target classes to high-risk jobs. Discuss ergonomic considerations in back pain prevention. Demonstrate back exercises.

 Set up a posture screening booth. Sponsor a safe-lifting clinic. Distribute material on back pain risk factor screening.

 Present the medical perspectives on back pain—address the question of when chiropractic care might be appropriate.

58 Be Sweet to Your Heart

Focus on heart disease during National Heart Month.

February is National Heart Month, usually a very big month for health promotion programs. This is a time when any program that relates to heart disease can be offered. Here are some useful ideas.

Starting Point

Contact the American Heart Association (see appendix) for current supporting materials and to find out what your local state chapters are doing that you might participate in. There will often be media coverage for these events that will give them increased visibility.

Tips for Success

- Plan activities that incorporate traditional heart disease and hypertension activities. (See Promotions 60 and 71.)
- Use themes associated with the month of February and Valentine's Day. (See Promotion 67.)
- This is a particularly good time to hold formal cholesterol and blood pressure screenings.
- Use valentine graphics with your promotional materials.

59 *Be Thankful for Your Health*

An opportunity for several programs linked to Thanksgiving.

Most people with good health would agree that it is something for which to be thankful. Use this theme as an entry into the difficult holiday season. Try some of the following.

Starting Point

Solicit Thanksgiving messages emphasizing success stories that participants are willing to share. Publish them in your newsletter or other communication. Tie the activity to other seasonal concepts such as Healthy Recipes for Thanksgiving or Great American Smokeout activities.

Tips for Success

- See the following promotions for ideas—*Weighting for the New Year* (Promotion #40, chapter 6), *Astrology Themes* (Promotion #56, chapter 9), *Healthy Holiday Gift Giving* (Promotion #64, chapter 9), or *Holiday Humbug* (Promotion #65, chapter 9).

60 *Blood Pressure Buddy System*

An inexpensive way of assuring that concerned employees receive regular checkups.

Organize this activity to promote self-care for hypertension prevention and control. Use the results of other blood pressure promotions or your health risk assessment screening to determine a target group. Here are some options.

Starting Point

 Hold a seminar featuring hypertension information. Follow up with a workshop instructing participants on how to take an accurate blood pressure reading. Encourage employees to form partnerships and register together for the activity. Distribute appropriate logs for tracking the readings. Encourage partners to take each other's blood pressure on a weekly basis.

Tips for Success

- Provide stethoscopes and manometers in convenient and secure locations accessible to participants.
- Offer incentives for those who take readings for a specified target number of consecutive weeks.
- Of course, activities such as this may require approval from your organization's medical advisor.
- Appropriate participant waivers may also be required by your legal advisor.
- A variation is to offer self-testing blood pressure devices and operate on an individual basis.

61 *Discover the New World*

A Columbus Day program to introduce nonparticipants to a new world of health through your program.

Columbus Day, October 12, may not be a major holiday to most people, but it presents an opportunity to promote your program to nonparticipants through a theme based on the discovery of a new world of health. Here are a few ideas on which you can build.

Starting Point

 Conduct an exercise journey from wherever your facility is to San Salvador, the probable site of the landing of Christopher Columbus. Since the distance will probably be significant, organize appropriately sized groups into crews of the three ships, the Niña, the Pinta, and the Santa María. Provide brief orientation sessions with an emphasis on discovering a new, healthier lifestyle. Emphasize the concept of discovering information about one's health through a personal testing series. Offer traditional fitness testing to new participants during the week in which Columbus Day falls. Use this as a springboard for your scheduled interventions.

Tips for Success

- Send personal invitations to nonparticipants.
- If your program is mature, most nonparticipants will probably be from the highest-risk and most-resistant groups. Plan some program activities geared specifically to this population.
- Include basic information and low-commitment activities.
- Keep the duration short and provide reinforcement for minimal participation by these important target employees.

62 *For Your Benefit*

*Give your program a boost during the benefits open
enrollment periods.*

Integration into the day-to-day operations of your organization is
one of the signs of a mature and successful program. Since health
promotion is often part of a benefits package, and since health promotion staff are generally good at communications, consider giving
your program added visibility and credibility by participating in your
organization's annual open enrollment. Here are some ideas for giving your program a boost.

Starting Point

Sponsor a financial planning seminar designed to help employees understand and maximize their pension, social security, and
401(K) plans. Schedule a series of brief (15 minutes) brown-bag
luncheons with program updates. Work with your benefits or
human resources department to design a set of simple calculations
that illustrate the cost benefit to an individual who chooses to stay
healthy.

Tips for Success

- Include incentives for enrollment in current program activities.
- Get involved in the early stages of planning the open enrollment. Be sure that your program has a prominent position in
  appropriate publications.
- Purchase self-care books to be distributed to employees. Provide them either as free gifts or as subsidized purchases. Ask the
  human resources or benefits department to cosponsor this promotion.

63 *Fresh Start*

Bring your program dropouts back at this traditional time of renewal.

Spring is a time of renewal. Use this theme as an opportunity to bring back your program dropouts. Here are some possibilities.

Starting Point

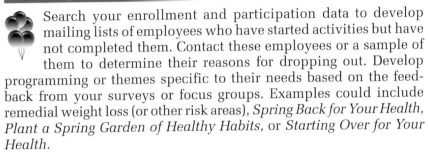

Search your enrollment and participation data to develop mailing lists of employees who have started activities but have not completed them. Contact these employees or a sample of them to determine their reasons for dropping out. Develop programming or themes specific to their needs based on the feedback from your surveys or focus groups. Examples could include remedial weight loss (or other risk areas), *Spring Back for Your Health, Plant a Spring Garden of Healthy Habits,* or *Starting Over for Your Health.*

Tips for Success

- Modify activities to meet the needs of this group with very modest goals and small incentives for intermediate goal achievement.
- Offer activities open only to dropouts.
- Kick off the activities or promotion on or about the vernal equinox in March.
- Attempt to transition into a summer program that builds on this effort.

64 *Healthy Holiday Gift Giving*

*Share the latest in holiday gifts that can enhance the health of
your employees' loved ones.*

Holiday gift giving is common to participants of most religious backgrounds. This can be an effective time to bring the health promotion messages you deliver at the workplace to friends and family. Share the latest in holiday gifts that can enhance the health of your employees' loved ones with some of these ideas.

Starting Point

 Prepare a catalog listing gift items, prices, and locations where they can be purchased. Or write a feature article on this topic for your employee newsletter. Include your catalog or a telephone number to order one.

Purchase or borrow gift items from the retailers and put them on display in a cafeteria or lobby. Bring the display to dispersed facilities that are large enough to justify it. Or set up the display in your office area and invite participants to drop by to see it. Hold a drawing for one or more of the items with participants registering as they view the display.

Tips for Success

- Research local retailers for the latest health-related gifts. Include as many risk areas as possible. Because of the abundance of fitness-related items, it is easy to overemphasize fitness. Include clothing, books, healthy cooking ideas, relaxation tapes, and so forth. Include items at a variety of prices. Try to negotiate discounts on behalf of your program.
- Work with local retailers who are having sales or promotions. They will often be very willing to work with you in exchange for the exposure to your participants.

65 *Holiday Humbug*

Explode common health myths with a brown-bag luncheon series.

One of the challenges you may be facing is the misinformation your participants have been exposed to over the years. It is human nature to take the path of least resistance, especially when faced with difficult changes. Quick fixes, magic pills, and special equipment are among a myriad of unproved or simply unwise approaches to behavior change that you should avoid. Misinformation must be unlearned before more sound approaches can be adopted. Consider exploding common health myths with a brown-bag luncheon series. Here is a list of topics to help you start.

Starting Point

 Develop a series with the following topics in mind: vitamin supplements, passive exercise equipment, cellulite reduction with skin creams, quackery in the 90s, organic foods, spot reducing, fad exercise equipment, or passive activities such as tai chi.

66 *New Year's Resolution Bulletin Board*

Help your employees stick to their resolutions while adding to your program participation.

New Year's is traditionally a time for your employees to make commitments to change. They make resolutions to lose weight, exercise, save money, or any of dozens of other sincere, well-meaning changes. The strength of these resolutions is that they occur at an opportune time, following the holiday party season, and they usually are spoken to others. The problem, however, is that when the process of change becomes difficult, they can easily drop out. Help your employees stick to their resolutions and succeed in their commitments to change while adding to your program participation by offering a system of support.

Starting Point

 Ask your participants to fill out an index card with their health-related resolution on one side and their name, address, and phone number on the other side. Develop a list from the data on the cards. Post the resolutions on a bulletin board (they should be in a secured bulletin board under glass to protect their confidentiality). Take the cards down after a week or two and store them for future use. Post them again after about six weeks to remind people about their commitments. Take the cards down after a week and store them again. After another four to six weeks, mail the cards back to their owners along with current promotional materials to support their changes.

Tips for Success

- If participation is low, plant some seeds by adding some of your own made-up resolutions to the display.
- Send appropriate promotional materials to participants based on their specific resolutions. Include basic informational pamphlets, public-domain brochures, and materials you have produced for program promotions. Promote classes, group activities, and brown-bag luncheons that have been planned around this event.
- Make a personal contact with each participant to remind them of their resolutions and offer your support after the second posting of the resolution cards.

67 *Sweetheart Seminar Series*

Explore ways that couples can help each other in the fight against heart disease.

One aspect of health promotion that is an ongoing challenge is the appropriate involvement of spouses or partners, on their own behalf or in support of their partners. Use the sweetheart theme to promote a seminar series designed to educate them on appropriate topics that could involve both partners. Here are some possibilities.

Starting Point

 Consider some of the following topics for your seminar series: sex after heart attacks, the role of aspirin in preventing heart attacks, estrogen therapy and heart attacks, food shopping as a heart attack prevention strategy, and CPR certification.

68 *The Heat Is On*

A summer safety program exploring summer issues related to the heat and sun.

Each year, more people die due to heat-related causes than cold-related causes. Give your employees the information they need to avoid danger for themselves and their families with a seminar series.

Starting Point

 Here are some possible topics for your seminar: heat-related first aid, heat-induced health conditions, heat dangers for the elderly, exercising or working in heat, avoiding dehydration, electrolyte replenishment during exercise, and nutritional considerations during heat.

69 *Veterans Day Celebration*

Honor the veterans of your program.

Veterans Day is celebrated nationally on November 11. Piggyback on the media promotion and public awareness of this date by honoring the veterans of your program. Be sensitive to the true meaning of the day and respectful of the war veterans while you also honor participants who have been faithful to your program's mission. Try some of these ideas.

Starting Point

Hold a *Show Your Shirt Day* when all participants who have earned one of your T-shirts wears the shirt either to work for the day or during a designated time such as lunch. This is particularly impressive if all of management is seen wearing earned T-shirts with their business attire.

If you work in an office complex with open office systems, especially a large open cubicle setting, try a *Balloon Day*. Attach helium-filled balloons to an object in the cubicle of each employee who has been involved in the program. The room will be filled with colorful balloons, reinforcing the popularity of the program to those who haven't yet joined.

Honor specific employees (with their permission) who have made significant lifestyle changes with a bulletin board display. Post their pictures and success stories on this Wall of Fame. Arrange for preferred parking privileges for the day for these honorees.

Tips for Success

- Consider honoring an employee of the week or month on an ongoing basis after kicking the event off on Veterans Day.

CHAPTER 10

General Promotional Ideas

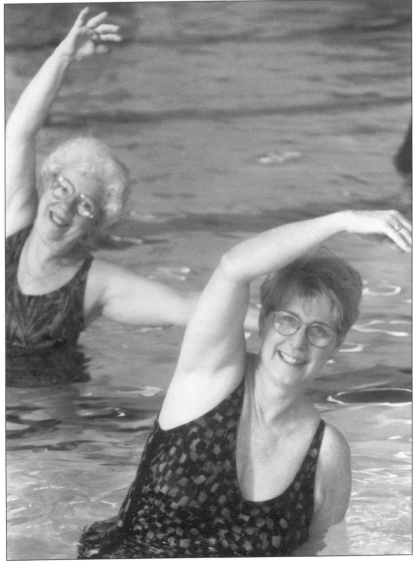

© Terry Wild Studio

70   *"Ask the Doc" Column*

Another feature for your newsletter.

In an era where medical self-care is becoming increasingly emphasized as an important part of managing costs, getting accurate information to employees is becoming more important. One way of doing this is with an *Ask the Doc* column in your newsletter.

Starting Point

Solicit the cooperation of an appropriate physician. Possibilities include the company medical director, a primary care physician from your HMO, a medical doctor from your health insurance carrier, or a physician within the community interested in getting positive exposure to build his or her practice. Write the column in a question and answer format. At the end of each column provide instructions on how to submit questions.

Tips for Success

- Begin the column with some seed questions that will be of general interest based on your knowledge of the population.
- Ask that names be given when possible so that if an urgency is detected, the individual can be contacted personally when appropriate.
- Keep a supply of your seed questions available in case interest wanes for a time.

71 *Birthday Blood Pressure*

A system that encourages regular monitoring of blood pressure for your employees.

Everyone should know their blood pressure. They especially need to know how it tracks over time. One way to provide this information is to use birthdays or another anniversary as a reminder for a blood pressure check.

Starting Point

 Use either a computer program or a file card system to organize the data. Each record should contain the following:
- Birth or anniversary date
- Name, address, and phone number of the employee
- Any specific information about the employee's blood pressure
- A log to record the annual reading that includes space to record readings of walk-ins
- Information about referrals made for abnormal readings

On or about the reminder date, send a card, e-mail, or fax to the employees. Ask them to come in for a reading within a week of receiving the reminder. If your program is structured so that appointments are needed, provide an easy way to make the appointment. As employees come in, take the readings; record the data; and provide information, counseling, or referrals to their health care providers as appropriate.

Tips for Success

- Be sure to use only trained staff and follow current blood pressure protocols.
- Use either the individual's birthday or the anniversary of their first day of employment as the reminder date.
- Solicit a general sign-up for the program in advance.
- Enroll all new employees as they begin with the organization.

72 *Congratulations Cards*

Build grassroots awareness throughout your organization.

One key to successful lifestyle change is to make a series of small positive changes rather than one huge dramatic change. Unfortunately these small changes often go unnoticed and therefore unrewarded. Here is a simple way to reinforce these health habits and also increase grassroots awareness.

Starting Point

 Print a series of wallet-sized cards with a brief message acknowledging the practice of healthy habits. For example, "Congratulations, you have been caught in the act of a healthy behavior." Include brief instructions on the card.

Tips for Success

- Instructions: If you spot a person practicing a healthy behavior, give them the card with an explanation of what you noticed. The behavior can be as simple as choosing a low-fat dressing in the cafeteria, parking at the far end of the parking lot, climbing the stairs rather than taking an elevator, or promoting humor by telling an appropriate joke. Inform the recipients that they should look for others practicing good health, especially those in apparent need of support. Ask them to hand the card off within two days.
- Enlist some of your key supporters or management to begin the congratulations process.
- Encourage the use of the cards by employees who travel to other facilities so recipients will notice the widespread acceptance of the program when they see the origination point of the card.
- If you have multiple facilities, print the name of the "home" facility for that card and the date of issue.

73 *Elevator Resource Center*

A different approach to providing information to employees in skyscrapers.

If you provide services in a multistory building with an elevator system, you can take advantage of the situation to bring program and promotional materials to employees who are not likely to come to your office. This idea will require permission from your facilities management, but is easy to implement after that.

Starting Point

Obtain a suitable portable cart on which to organize promotional materials. At the publicized time, post "out of order" signs on the doors to the elevator shaft you will be using and bring one elevator with your materials cart to the designated floor and lock it on that floor until the schedule calls for a move to another floor. Move the elevator to the new floor at each scheduled time.

Tips for Success

- Monitor the elevator usage informally and poll employees to determine whether the project is causing inconvenience in elevator access. If it is, either modify the schedule, or cancel it.
- Determine an appropriate schedule for each floor of the building. Be consistent in the schedule and publicize it. Be sure not to schedule the elevator for your use during peak usage times.

Extended Campus Classes

An alternative to traditional education that may help with commuter populations.

Attending educational classes during lunch or after work may be difficult or impossible for employees who have certain jobs, are in carpools, or have small children or other obligations. Consider using other community resources to offer "extended campus" classes.

Starting Point

 Make arrangements with your instructors or vendors to teach at the selected locations (such as a local recreation center). In many cases you can use a facility without cost, especially if the general public may also participate in the classes. This might work especially well in small communities.

Tips for Success

- Possible locations include school gyms, classrooms, auditoriums or libraries; church basements or meeting rooms; bank or chamber-of-commerce meeting rooms; shopping mall community rooms; and movie theaters during off-hours.
- If getting sufficient numbers of employees to register and attend is a problem, consider forming an alliance with another local business facing the same problem. They may have facilities that can be shared.

75 *House Calls*

A bold approach in gaining management support.

Often management staff is reluctant to participate in program activities for a variety of reasons. One solution to their failure to participate is to eliminate as many excuses as possible by bringing the activity to them in their offices. Here's one approach.

Starting Point

 Equip an appropriate staff member or yourself with a black bag. In the black bag place a manometer, stethoscope, and appropriate educational materials. Create a blood pressure log on a Rolodex file card to be filed in the letter B section of the manager's Rolodex. Show up at the offices of your management staff. Consider showing up unannounced, as many of these individuals do not take the time to plan to participate. However, be sensitive to your political environment and consult with human resources before showing up unannounced. If you are advised against it make brief (less than ten-minute) appointments. Offer a free blood pressure check in the privacy of their office.

Tips for Success

- Use the time while you are pumping up the manometer and asking the manager to rest briefly before the reading to pass along appropriate information about the program or blood pressure. Be sensitive to how the manager is receiving this unsolicited interaction and don't wear out your welcome.
- Offer to drop in for monthly readings and use this as a springboard to a supportive relationship.

76 *Limited Space Health Fair*

A system for health fairs that will work anywhere.

Health fairs are a staple in the health promotion field. They come in all shapes and sizes and can add a great deal of visibility to any program. However, in many settings a traditional health fair won't work because of space and time: It is usually conducted in a single large space such as a cafeteria, and often over a relatively short time period such as one lunch shift of one to two hours. If this formula doesn't work for you, try the following approach.

Starting Point

Create and prioritize a list of all those resources that seem appropriate to feature in health fair booths. Plan displays to meet your program objectives. Find space and proceed with scheduling exhibitors and vendors. Finally assign booths. Create a suggested walking tour of all the exhibits allowing employees to begin anywhere on the route. Don't forget to produce appropriate signs to keep your health fair moving!

Tips for Success

- Plan on using internal and external resources to promote various program components.
- Contact the appropriate individuals in management who have the authority to grant you the use of these spaces for a health fair. Find out who controls the reservation of the space and what those procedures are.
- Do a survey of your physical facility to identify every location that could support a booth. Plot all of the available spaces on a map of the building. Record locations of electrical outlets, access, and safety considerations such as fire escapes, extinguishers, and so forth. Be sure that spaces such as dead-end hallways do not violate fire codes when used in this manner. Based on the results of your physical survey, match your prioritized list of exhibits with the survey to determine a "short list."
- Look for dead-end hallways, conference rooms of any size, small break rooms, any available portion of the cafeteria, lobby space, waiting areas, and outdoor spaces.

- Numbering the stations makes getting through the fair easier.
- Hold the fair over break periods, lunch, and before and after work to allow employees to piece together an entire tour of the fair if they don't have a large enough block of available personal time.
- Hold drawings at the end of the fair for prizes. Do not require that employees be present to win, as this would merely be another obstacle to participation.
- Promote an exercise walking tour of the various locations with a measured walking path with maps and clear signs.
- Use standard health fair planning logistics for maximizing promotion, including bingo or punch cards; fishbowl drawings; special incentives for signing up for activities (in order to develop mailing lists for follow-up); free handouts, gifts, or incentives at all stations; and shopping bags to carry incentive items.

77 *Placemats With Tear-Off Registrations*

Another way of making registrations easy.

Convincing employees to participate in activities that require registration is essentially the same as a sales process. The product is the activity, the customer is the employee, the price is their time and/or a modest copayment. Anything that prevents them from "buying" is an objection that must be overcome by you, the salesperson. Here's a simple idea to make registration for any event easy.

Starting Point

Develop standard table tents promoting the event. If you have a cafeteria that uses plastic trays, get the exact measurements of the trays and design a placemat to fit. Design the upper part of the placemat to include the essential information about the event. Be sure to include your logo or other program identity. Design the lower part to be a tear-off registration form.

Tips for Success

- Be sure a pencil is available at all tables. You may have to tie them down or replace them frequently.
- Provide drop boxes at all entrances and exits to the cafeteria as well as at cashier locations. Empty them daily.

78 *Posting Network*

Gain leverage by using existing staff to help reach dispersed populations.

Communications is a constant challenge in any health promotion program, but especially in one with multiple locations. While every employee is entitled to full participation in the program, it simply is not cost-effective to expect a personal on-site presence at small, remote locations. However, conventional communications methods such as flyers and bulletin boards are still effective. A posting network is a basic health promotion strategy for programs with multiple locations that gives you leverage for your labor. Here's how to put it together.

Starting Point

Identify one key individual within each target building to be your network member. This person should have authority to maintain bulletin boards, access to copy machines, and of course an interest in the program. Develop a distribution list or preprint labels for all locations. Instruct network members on the posting procedures:

- Postings should go up within 24 hours of receiving the master copy.
- Multiple copies should be made if more than one location is to be posted.
- Take-down dates, which should be printed on every flyer, should be strictly adhered to.
- Prepare clean copies on white paper for distribution to the network.

This system works very well for any of the commercially available camera-ready flyers if you can add site-specific information.

Tips for Success

- Be sure the copies include all appropriate information and a number to call for more information. Do not expect or rely on the network person to be able to provide program information.
- This system can also be used for maintaining "take-one" boxes.

- If possible, try to make occasional personal contact at these locations if your time and the size and location of the facility permits.
- Master copies of handouts should also be available when appropriate.

79 *Stay Safe Saloon*

Be part of a holiday safe driving campaign.

Many communities and organizations participate in safe driving and responsible holiday hosting campaigns in an effort to reduce drunk driving over the holidays. Here is a simple idea that can be part of a holiday campaign.

Starting Point

Obtain as many recipes for nonalcoholic holiday drinks as you can find. Sources include soft drink and juice companies, state safety councils, MADD chapters, and state highway patrol public affairs officers. You can also use a variety of cookbooks that are available in most bookstores or the local library. Select no more than six of these beverages for use in the event. Prepare the drinks and provide small, sample-sized paper cups for sampling. Serve the beverages over the lunch period and provide handouts with the following: copies of all of the recipes being sampled, responsible holiday hosting ideas, designated driver promotion, taxi reimbursement information if your organization or community provides it, and other safe winter driving tips if they apply in your location.

Tips for Success

- Prepare a display for the Monthly Minute. It can be as simple as a decorated table top, or as elaborate as a set of swinging doors with a saloon motif.
- Combine the event with (or use the event to promote) other safe driving campaign activities that are planned.

80   *Support Groups*

Strengthen one of the weak links in health promotion.

One component that is often either missing or de-emphasized in health promotion programs is that of support or maintenance after behavior changes have been established. Here are some easy ways to establish support groups for your employees.

Starting Point

Establish the need through surveys and focus groups. Create a mailing list for targeted individuals that you have discovered through any appropriate means. Publicize the group and establish an initial meeting time, date, and place. Arrange for a content expert to be present at the initial meeting (who may also be available at future meetings on an as-needed basis). At the meeting, introduce your expert, determine the goals of the group, and share your own. Identify potential group leaders who can assist in communications and logistics as well as possibly assisting with discussion. Formally leading a group may be inappropriate for an untrained person, and if so, your expert may be needed on a regular basis.

Tips for Success

- Possible areas for ongoing support groups include: weight control, smoking cessation, postcardiac-event recovery, Alcoholics Anonymous, postdivorce, single parents, sandwich generation or elder care issues, Alzheimer's disease, parents of teenage children, survivor syndrome (after workforce reductions), and hypertension.
- Establish a proposed meeting schedule and use your connections to reserve rooms and obtain management permission if needed.
- Attend occasional meetings yourself to keep in touch with their activities and status.
- Promote the groups generally as well as specifically when they need a boost.
- Consider the groups one of your available resources for at-risk individuals, especially after your primary interventions.

81 *Top Ten Excuses T-Shirt Contest*

Focus on rejuvenating your backsliders and program dropouts in a lighthearted way.

Try this activity to give a boost to any existing program with a focus on bringing employees who did not have success back for additional work.

Starting Point

Announce and promote the contest well in advance of your proposed activity kickoff. Ask participants to submit their best excuse for why they did not succeed in meeting their health behavior change goals. Ask for two excuses—one that was a legitimate problem for them and another humorous excuse. Have the excuses judged by your employee wellness committee or other staff. Offer support, guidance, or suggestions on how to overcome the legitimate excuses for all entrants. Use the humorous excuses for the contest.

Tips for Success

- Order your T-shirts with the "Top Ten Excuses" printed on the shirt.
- Award a free T-shirt to the employees who submitted the selected ten excuses.
- Use the list of entrants as a targeted mailing list for promotion of the activities of interest to each individual.

82   *Voucher Systems*

*Another way of helping dispersed populations to participate in
your program.*

In large organizations, there is often a disparity in program offer-
ings between large central locations and smaller remote locations.
One way of providing at least some health promotion service is
through the use of voucher systems to encourage participation in the
program and a feeling of belonging. Make participation in your health
risk appraisal process a prerequisite for obtaining vouchers for other
aspects of the program such as a community-based education program. Try some of these ideas.

Starting Point

 Determine what your average cost per participant (rather than
per eligible employee) is for a typical 12-month period. Use
this figure as a starting point to calculate a figure to be considered a maximum total annual allocation to remote individuals
who apply for program voucher funding. The allocation can be distributed through expense report/reimbursement systems, vouchers
that the organization will redeem for a cash payment, or direct payment to vendors who have a master agreement to provide services to
employees. Make some decisions about what activities will be al-
lowed under the voucher program for either full or partial payment.
Examples include registration fees for a smoking cessation program
that has been approved, blood tests as a stand-alone screening activity or as part of a health risk assessment screening component, subscriptions to approved health-related magazines, membership fees
to approved community-based fitness centers or health clubs, and
other activities that support achievement of program goals.

Tips for Success

- Consider increasing the total annual allocation to compensate
  for the additional cost to deliver services without the advantage
  of high volume centralized activities.
- Consider decreasing the total annual allocation to compensate
  for fixed costs such as labor and rent.
- In a corporate setting, you will have to work closely with your ac-
  counting department, benefits department, and human resources to
  assure compliance with applicable laws and organizational policies.

83 *Wellness Grants*

Fund grassroots projects through this grant system.

Grassroots support can be a valuable key to long-term success in health promotion. It is often difficult, however, to gain this support in remote or small facilities that do not receive the benefits of the full range of programming available to larger, centrally located sites. One way of improving this situation is through a system of wellness grants. Wellness grants are financial grants that can be allocated to departments, buildings, or special-interest groups to create additional opportunities related to improving employees' physical health. They are not intended for use by individuals. An example would be the purchase of a refrigerator to allow a small site to bring in healthier foods than may be offered through a vending machine. Here's how to set a system up.

Starting Point

 Establish a source of funding to begin the project. Sources include a line item in your annual budget request, a special line item in another budget such as that of the benefits department, a special allocation from a senior executive, or proceeds from special fund-raising activities. Next, establish protocols for an application process. These should be as simple as possible while still providing adequate information and justification. Then establish a review committee with representation from employees and management as well as you or your staff. Define their roles and responsibilities, meeting frequency, and tenure. Establish criteria to help the committee in their approval process. Discuss the criteria and, if possible, an objective rating system for each criteria. Be sure to let the employees know that only a finite amount of grant money is available and that projects that are not funded can be resubmitted in the future.

Tips for Success

- Before finalizing the project, you will need to get some assurance that future funding is likely.
- Possible criteria include size of the request; number of employees who will benefit from the request; evidence of grassroots support; consistency with the program's mission statement, goals,

and objectives; miscellaneous concerns such as liability, probability of success, and probability of longevity; amount of maintenance, labor, or future support required for success; evaluation and reporting mechanisms; and relative need in terms of the amount of attention and other resources the program has given to the site in the past (that is, a sorely neglected location may be given preference).

- Promote the concept to employees, encouraging them to apply for projects like exercise mats for aerobic exercise classes or a fitness center with a bike and treadmill. Other examples include outdoor fitness equipment such as basketball hoops, a bark chip walking path, or bike racks; or other health-related materials like a library resource center or special-interest literature or subscriptions.

84 Your Health Is in Your Hands

A program to increase awareness of prevention of the common cold in time for the cold season.

Here is a Monthly Minute designed to increase awareness of prevention of the common cold and other communicable diseases in time for the cold season. Plan this one for late fall when colds are just beginning to go around.

Starting Point

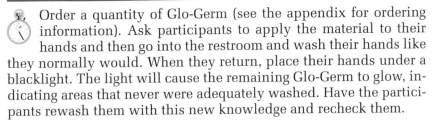 Order a quantity of Glo-Germ (see the appendix for ordering information). Ask participants to apply the material to their hands and then go into the restroom and wash their hands like they normally would. When they return, place their hands under a blacklight. The light will cause the remaining Glo-Germ to glow, indicating areas that never were adequately washed. Have the participants rewash them with this new knowledge and recheck them.

Tips for Success

- Handouts should give information about the spread of the common cold and other communicable diseases.
- This event is also very compatible with the distribution of other self-care health materials.

Resources

As you go about the business of health promotion, you will have a wealth of valuable assistance in the form of public, private, non-profit, and for-profit resources. These include government agencies, private organizations, and professional associations. The list given here is not intended to be exhaustive. The inclusion of an organization does not constitute an endorsement. They are listed to give you a starting point from which to network into resources that may meet your program's needs. Begin to build your own database of other resources and to assemble files with materials that you gather from any source.

Government Agencies

Many organizations that are funded by the federal, state, or local government have information, materials, and even human resources that will be useful in creating and implementing program ideas. Most of their services are free or low-cost.

United States

The Centers for Disease Control and Prevention (CDC)
1600 Clifton Road NE
Atlanta, GA 30333
Phone: 404-639-3311
Web address: http://www.cdc.gov/
  A source for publications, health information, data, and statistics.

Food and Drug Administration (FDA)
Office of Consumer Affairs
FDA/HFE-88, 5600 Fishers Lane
Rockville, MD 20857
Phone: 301-443-3170
Fax: 301-443-9767
Web address: http://www.fda.gov/
  Consumer education on health, drugs, and nutrition.   **125**

The National Institutes of Health (NIH)
Bethesda, MD 20892
Web address: http://www.nih.gov/

Data, statistics, and research on a wide variety of health issues.

United States Department of Agriculture (USDA)
1200 Jefferson Drive
Washington, DC 20250
Phone: 202-720-2791
Fax: 202-720-2166
Web address: http://www.usda.gov/
For a listing of programs at the state level:
http://www.reeusda.gov/hew/statepartners/usa.htm

Provides educational materials and programs, especially on nutrition and consumer issues.

State Health Departments

State health departments often have educational materials and programs available. Services and expertise will vary from state to state. Consult your local phone book for specific resources.

County Health Agencies

Most counties have active extension services that offer community outreach services on health-related topics. These often include both education and health screening services. Consult your local phone book for specific resources.

Nonprofit Organizations

Nonprofit organizations offer free and inexpensive health education materials as well as local in-person resources. They frequently will exhibit at health fairs and can provide speakers and educational programs.

Alcoholics Anonymous
475 Riverside Drive
New York, NY 10015
Phone: 212-870-3400
Fax: 212-870-3003
Web address: http://www.alcoholics-anonymous.org/

American Cancer Society
1599 Clifton Road NE
Atlanta, GA 30329-4251
Office phone: 404-320-3333
Library phone: 404-329-9780
E-mail: Library@cancer.org
Web address: http://www.cancer.org

Provides materials and programs on all aspects of cancer screening and prevention. A primary resource for the Great American Smokeout.

American Diabetes Association
1660 Duke Street
Alexandria, VA 22314
Phone: 800-232-3472
Fax: 703-549-6995
Web address: http://www.diabetes.org

Materials and programs specific to diabetes.

American Heart Association
7272 Greenville Avenue
Dallas, TX 75231-4596
Phone: 214-706-1521
Fax: 214-952-4334
E-mail: inquire@amhrt.org
Web address: http://www.amhrt.org/ahawho.htm

Programs and materials on heart disease, hypertension, cholesterol, and related topics. Provides training and certification for blood pressure reading.

American Kidney Fund
6110 Executive Boulevard
Rockville, MD 20852
Phone: 800-638-8299
Fax: 301-881-0898
E-mail: helplinen@akfinc.org
Web address: http://www.arbon.com/kidney

Materials and programs related to kidney diseases. A primary source of information on organ donation.

American Lung Association
1740 Broadway
New York, NY 10019-4374
Phone: 212-315-8700
Fax: 212-265-5642
E-mail: info@lungusa.org
Web address: http://www.lungusa.org

Materials and programs related to lung diseases.

Harvard Health Publications Group
164 Longwood Avenue
Boston, MA 02115
Phone: 617-432-1485
Fax: 617-432-1506
Web address: http://www.med.harvard.edu/publications/
Health_Publications/index.html

Publishers of monthly consumer newsletters including Harvard Health Letter, Harvard Women's Health Watch, Harvard Men's Health Watch, Harvard Heart Letter, Harvard Mental Health Letter, *and* Digestive Health and Nutrition.

March of Dimes
1275 Mamaroneck
White Plains, NY 10605
Phone: 914-428-7100
E-mail: worksiteprog@modimes.org
Web address: http://modimes.org

Program assistance, particularly in the area of prenatal care and prevention of birth defects and low-birthweight babies.

National American Red Cross
8111 Gatehouse Road
Falls Church, VA 22042
Phone: 703-206-6000
Fax: 703-206-7673
Web address: http://www.redcross.org/hss

A wide variety of programs, including water safety and blood donation.

National Institute for Fitness and Sport
250 University Boulevard
Indianapolis, IN 46202-5192
Phone: 317-274-3432
Fax: 317-274-7408

Educational programs and materials. Other on-site services in the Indianapolis area.

National Wellness Institute
1300 College Court
Stevens Point, WI 54481
Phone: 715-342-2969
Fax: 715-342-2979
E-mail: nwi@wellnessnwi.org
Web address: http://www.wellnesswni.org/

A source for materials and networking with other resources.

Park Nicollet *HealthSource*
3800 Park Nicollet Boulevard
Minneapolis, MN 55416
Phone: 612-993-3534

Worksite services, health promotion publications, and personal fitness services.

Wellness Councils of America (WELCOA)
Community Health Plaza
Suite 311
7101 Newport Avenue
Omaha, NE 68152-2100
Phone: 402-572-3590

Provides predesigned activities, incentive programs, and materials. State-level councils available in many states. Good networking opportunities at the state level.

World Health Organization
CH-12N Geneva 27
Switzerland
Phone: +41 22 791 2111
Fax: +41 22 791 0746
E-mail: postmaster@who.ch
Web address: http://www.who.ch/welcome/html

> *An international resource for information on a broad range of health-related topics.*

YMCA of the USA
101 North Wacker Drive
Chicago, IL 60606-7386
Phone: 312-977-0031
Fax: 312-977-9063
Web address: See http://www.tasd.edu.au/tasonline/ymca/www-usa.htm for a listing of YMCAs across the country.

> *Can be a source of educational programs, and both on- and off-site fitness programs.*

For-Profit Organizations

While the primary intent of this book is to provide inexpensive program ideas, sometimes it is more cost-effective to outsource a specific program or function. Whether to outsource or handle a function yourself will depend on your time, talents, and budget. Here are some well-known for-profit organizations that may offer something you need. Their inclusion is not an endorsement of their products or services.

Amazon.com Books
Phone: 800-201-7575
E-Mail: info@amazon.com
http://www.amazon.com/exec/obidos/isbn%sd0809233614/2148-5244337-092750

> *Source for* Chase's Calendar of Events, *an extensive listing of unique and familiar events associated with every day, week, and month of the year. Useful for clever promotional event planning. Ordering through this vendor is on-line only.*

American Corporate Health Programs, Inc.
559 West Uwchlan Avenue
Suite 220
Exton, PA 19341
Phone: 610-594-2110
Fax: 610-594-9079

Provides program development, management, staffing, products, and services for health and fitness programming for on-site or dispersed groups. Also offers demand management and disease management programming and products.

American Institute for Preventive Medicine
30445 Northwestern Highway
Suite 350
Farmington Hills, MI 48334-3102
Phone: 800-345-2476; 810-539-1800
Fax: 810-539-1808
E-mail: aipm@healthy.net
Web address: http://aipm.healthy.net

Provides self-care publications, seminars, and health promotion programs that focus on demand management, smoking cessation, weight control, stress management, self-esteem enhancement, prenatal education, fitness, nutrition, and EAP.

Glo-Germ
P.O. Box 537
Moab, UT 84532
Phone: 800-842-6622
Fax: 801-259-5930
E-mail: moabking@sisna.com
Web address: http://www.glogerm.com/

Source for Glo-Germ as described in chapter 10.

Health Enhancement Systems
P.O. Box 1335
Midland, MI 48641-1335
Phone: 800-326-2317; 517-839-0852
Fax: 517-839-0025

Publisher of Health Promotion Practitioner *newsletter, a monthly idea source for health promoters and wellness program managers.*

Hope Publications
350 East Michigan Avenue
Suite 301
Kalamazoo, MI 49007-3851
Phone: 616-343-0770
Fax: 616-343-6260

Health-related newsletter and other publications.

Johnson and Johnson Health Care Systems, Inc.
425 Hoes Lane
Piscataway, NJ 08855
Phone: 800-443-3682
Fax: 908-562-2297

A wide range of health promotion products and services.

Krames Communications
1100 Grundy Lane
San Bruno, CA 94066-3030
Phone: 800-333-3032
Fax: 415-244-4512
Web address: http://www.krames.com

Health-related pamphlets, brochures, and educational materials.

National Wellness Speakers Bureau
3722 West 50th Street
Suite 110
Minneapolis, MN 55410
Phone: 612-925-4090
Fax: 612-925-2135
E-mail: wellspeak@aol.com

Provides speakers, seminars, and workshops.

Personal Best
420 5th Avenue South
Suite D
Edmonds, WA 98020
Phone: 800-888-7853

Fax: 206-775-8250

E-mail: info@personalbest.com

Publishers of health newsletters, including senior, low-literacy, and Spanish editions. Customization is available.

StayWell Health Management Systems

1340 Mendota Heights Road

St. Paul, MN 55120-1128

Phone: 612-454-3577

Fax: 612-454-4062

E-mail: marketing@staywell.com

Web address: http://www.mosbych.com

Offers health risk assessment and screening programs, health education for at-risk populations, health newsmagazine, and consulting and evaluation services.

Teraco Products

2080 Commerce Drive

Midland, TX 79703

Phone: 915-694-7736

Fax: 800-333-9694

E-mail: info@teraco.com

Manufacturers of Stress Cards and other plastic products. They do not sell direct but can direct you to a local distributor, usually a vendor of promotional products.

Weight Watchers International, Inc.

175 Crossways Park West

Woodbury, NY 11797

Phone: 800-651-6000

http://www.weight-watchers.com/

Individual and group weight-management programs, including on-site Weight Watchers at Work.

Whole Person Associates
(A division of Pfeifer-Hamilton Publishers)
210 West Michigan
Duluth, MN 55802-1908
Phone: 800-247-6789; 218-727-0500
Fax: 218-727-0505
E-mail: books@wholeperson.com
Web address: http://wholeperson.com/~books

> *Stress and wellness specialists offering professional development and personal growth resources for health professionals, counselors, trainers, consultants, educators, and group leaders. A source for stress dots.*

Professional Associations

Professional associations can be a rich source of ideas, including research conference opportunities, printed materials, and networking opportunities.

American College of Sports Medicine
P.O. Box 1440
Indianapolis, IN 46206-1440
Phone: 317-637-9200
Fax: 317-634-7817
E-mail: pipacsm@acsm.org
Web address: http://www.a1.com/sportsmed/

American Medical Association
515 North State Street
Chicago, IL 60610
Phone: 312-464-5000
Web address: http://www.ama-assn.org/

Association for Worksite Health Promotion (AWHP)
60 Revere Drive, Suite 500
Northbrook, IL 60062
Phone: 847-489-9574
Fax: 847-480-9282
E-mail: awhp@awhp.com
Web address: http://www.awhp.com/

Miscellaneous

A particularly interesting Internet Web site has been developed by Austin State University. It contains dozens of links to other health-related Web sites, including government agencies, associations, journals and other publications, and colleges and universities.

Austin State University
Web address: http://www.tahperd.sfasu.edu/links3.html

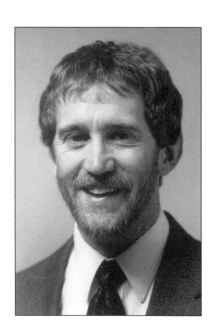

About the Author

Timothy Glaros is the owner of Creative Business Consulting and is the national sales manager for Ceridan Performance Partners' employee assistance and LifeBalance services. He specializes in program design, implementation, planning, promotional techniques, and internal marketing. In previous positions Glaros was a manager for Control Data's Stay Well program, which covered more than 25,000 employees in 14 major locations. In addition to being the coauthor of the book *Managing Health Promotion Programs,* Glaros has written numerous articles for such publications as *Health Education, Fitness in Business,* and *HK Magazine.* He has also given more than 80 presentations at conferences throughout the country.

Glaros received his master's degree in education from the University of Minnesota in 1975. Before entering the business world, he taught health and physical education in the Mounds View (Minnesota) Public Schools. Glaros has been an active member of Association for Worksite Health Promotion (AWHP) since 1983, serving as a regional president and being selected as a Fellow in 1991.

POINT LOMA NAZARENE UNIVERSITY
RYAN LIBRARY

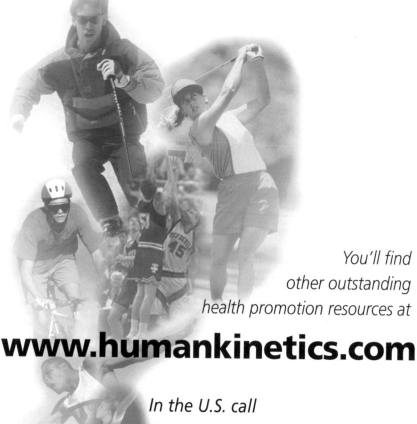

*You'll find
other outstanding
health promotion resources at*

www.humankinetics.com

In the U.S. call

1-800-747-4457

Australia ....(08) 8277-1555
Canada..............................(800) 465-7301
Europe .... +44 (0) 113-278-1708
New Zealand ....(09) 309-1890

HUMAN KINETICS
The Information Leader in Physical Activity
P.O. Box 5076 • Champaign, IL 61825-5076 USA